AF567185

Fu Qing-zhu's Gynecology

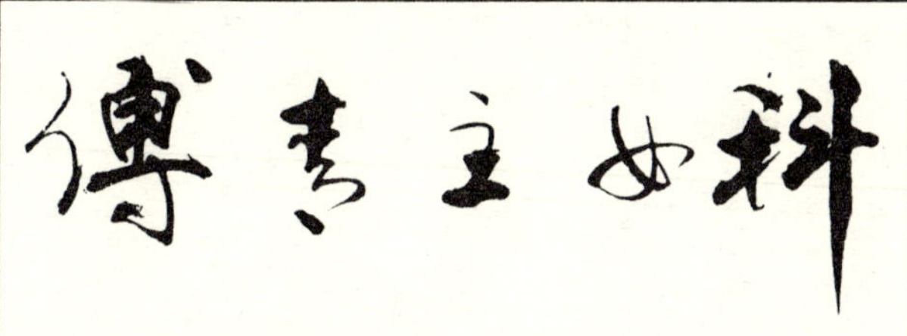

Fu Qing-zhu's Gynecology

translated by

Yang Shou-zhong & Liu Da-wei

BLUE POPPY PRESS

Published by:

BLUE POPPY PRESS
1775 LINDEN AVE.
BOULDER, CO 80304

FIRST EDITION
MAY 1992

Library of Congress #92-0712293
ISBN 0-936185-35-X

Printed at Westview Press, Boulder, CO
Cover Printed at D & K Printing, Boulder, CO

This book is printed on archive quality, acid free, recycled paper.

Editor's Preface

Several years ago, Dr. Ku Su-liang, director of the Florida College of Traditional Chinese Medicine, invited me to co-teach a workshop on TCM gynecology. Dr. Ku introduced the seminar with a history of traditional Chinese gynecology or *fu ke*. In his lecture, Dr. Ku mentioned *Fu Qing Zhu Nu Ke* or *Fu Qing-zhu's Gynecology*. I had read of Fu Qing-zhu and even owned a copy of part of his gynecology text (*Fo Shan Yi Xue Shou Gao [A Manuscript of Fo Shan's Medical Theories]*). But at that time, I knew little about Fu Qing-zhu or the import of his work. Dr. Ku mentioned that *Fu Qing Zhu Nu Ke* was one of *the* most important TCM gynecology books. He said that Fu Qing-zhu had not been content to merely paraphrase the classics and cite other TCM gynecologists before him. Dr. Ku also said that *Fu Qing-zhu's Gynecology* is the basis for many modern TCM gynecological theories, diagnoses, and prescriptions.

Attempting to specialize in the practice of TCM gynecology, Dr. Ku's remarks piqued my interest in learning what was contained in this famous gynecology book by Fu Qing-zhu. References to formulas by Fu Qing-zhu and quotes from his *Nu Ke* appearing in other, more modern TCM gynecology texts only further whet my appetite for this classic. When Cong Chun-yu, president of the Gansu College of Traditional Chinese Medicine who is also a *fu ke* specialist, sent me an article on the treatment of infertility in which every case was based on a section from *Fu Qing Zhu Nu Ke*, I knew I had to read this book one way or another. Although I have myself attempted to translate parts of *Fu Qing Zhu Nu Ke* for my own use and for inclusion in books of my own on TCM gynecology, I have never felt that I had either the time or the Chinese language skills to translate this classic in full.

A year or so ago, Yang Shou-zhong, an English language medical translator associated with the North China Coalmines Medical College in Tangshan, Hebei, People's Republic of China, wrote me asking if there were any Chinese medical books I might be interested in his translating for publication by Blue Poppy Press. I immediately sent him back a list of three books, Huang-fu Mi's *Zhen Jiu Jia Yi Jing*, Fu Qing-zhu's *Nu Ke*, and Li Dong-yuan's *Pi Wei Lun*. With my request in hand, Mr. Yang organized a translation group under his tutelage and direction and, in less than eighteen months, submitted to Blue Poppy working manuscripts of these three seminal Chinese medical classics. The following translation of *Fu Qing Zhu Nu Ke* is the first of this group to be published. Its publication inaugurates a new series of books by Blue Poppy Press, the Great Masters Series.

Although Yang Shou-zhong and his co-translator of this book, Liu Da-wei, have given an ample and interesting introduction to the life and works of Fu Qing-zhu, a.k.a. Fo Shan, there are a few things which need to be said regarding this book for its English-speaking readers. Though it is, indeed, one of the most important sources of TCM *fu ke* or gynecological theory and practice, as a premodern text, its diagnoses, theories, and treatments are but a record of one man's practice. As the reader will see, Fu Qing-zhu introduces almost each and every disease category by the remarks that, while most people think the disease under discussion is due to such and such a mechanism, he thinks it is really due to another disease mechanism. The unsuspecting reader might then infer that, for each disease, only a single mechanism exists, and this is not so.

One of the strong points of contemporary TCM is that it has gathered all the various theories and pattern discriminations for various diseases proposed by its most illustrious historical and contemporary practitioners and synthesized these in such a way that, under any given disease, all the possible patterns accompanying that disease are each described. Contemporary students of TCM are familiar with the fact that, under, let's say, *tong jing* or dysmenorrhea, there are a half dozen disease mechanisms and patterns, each with their discriminating signs and symptoms, tongue, and pulse, their own unique therapeutic principles, and their own guiding formulas. Today, such multi-pattern breakdowns are common for most diseases, be they traditional Chinese diseases or modern Western diseases. For most diseases, there are several different possible mechanisms for their arising, and, therefore, since TCM therapy aims to eradicate these root disease mechanisms and not just palliate their symptoms, each separate mechanism or pattern requires its own treatment. Therefore, treatment predicated on pattern discrimination or *bian zheng lun zhi* has become the *modus operandi* and hallmark of contemporary TCM.

One of the reasons that Fu Qing-zhu's *Nu Ke* is so important is that Fu Qing-zhu identified a number of patterns for gynecological diseases which previous authorities had overlooked. Many of the pattern discriminations in TCM gynecology which we now take for granted have their *locus classicus* in this book. That does not mean, however, that each of Fu Qing-zhu's discussions of individual disease categories is categorically complete. As I read his book, Fu Qing-zhu was interested in pointing out those places where, through his own clinical experience and insight, he had something to add to the already existing body of knowledge of his day. His book was not meant to be an exhaustive text on TCM gynecology giving each and every possible variation. Rather it is a record of the pith of what Fu Qing-zhu had to say in contradistinction to what everyone before had said on each *fu ke* or *nu ke* disease category.

Therefore, this book is not a comprehensive text on TCM gynecology. Nor are its discussions and treatment protocols categorically sufficient for the contemporary practice of TCM gynecology. Thus, it is not meant so much for the undergraduate TCM student as the experienced practitioner interested in further understanding the historical development of TCM *fu ke*. Such advanced TCM practitioners will find this book a gold mine of sophisticated TCM reason and logic. Readers following Fu Qing-zhu's syllogisms cannot help but be struck by the penetrating depth of his insight and the way he was able to cut to the quick of a problem. Nor can they fail to be struck by the elegant simplicity of his formulas and their rationales. Indeed, one of the hallmarks of Fu Qing-zhu's method is to achieve a certain therapeutic effect without actually using medicinals normally said to achieve that effect. In other words, Fu Qing-zhu often would stop bleeding without using *zhi xue* or stop bleeding medicinals, would stop vomiting without using *zhi ou* herbs, would promote lactation without using *tong ru* or lactation-promoting ingredients, etc.

As a TCM practitioner specializing in *fu ke* or gynecology, finally having access to Fu Qing-zhu's *Nu Ke* is like filling in a space on one's family tree. I can now read my predecessor's thoughts on this or that problem, appreciating his logic and the formula he prescribed. However, although this book helps to give me greater perspective on my art and craft, it also underscores how far TCM has come in its development since the early Qing Dynasty. Until only fairly recently, the history and practice of Chinese medicine was rife with sectarianism. Students of one teacher or adherents of one school jealously guarded their theories and techniques, seldom sharing these openly. When one thinks about the great efforts made in the People's Republic of China in the last 40 years to expand and unify the practice of TCM, one can only feel grateful for this endeavor. Though these efforts have sometimes gone to extremes, downplaying or eliminating certain theories or practices not congruent with the current political doctrines or social dogmas, they have, nonetheless, created a grand scheme which is at least as large as the sum of its parts.

As technical points, this translation is based on the 1978 edition published by the Shanghai People's Press. The material in parentheses has been added by the translators in order to make the English read more easily while at the same time conveying some of the flavor of the Chinese original. Material in brackets was added by some unspecified historical editor. Since these additions do, in many instances, add useful clinical information, we have decided to retain them. Medicinal ingredients are identified by latinate pharmacological nomenclature followed by the *pinyin* romanization of the Chinese name given in the text. The amounts of these ingredients is given in the traditional Chinese weights and measures found in the original. Typically today, 1 *qian* equals 3.125 grams, 1 *liang*, therefore, 31.25 grams, and 1 *fen*, 0.3125 grams. Formula names are given first in pinyin and then translated in parentheses. The English terminology used in this translation is largely based on Wiseman and Boss' *Glossary of Chinese Medical Terms and Acupuncture Points*. In a very few instances, we have chosen not to follow Wiseman and Boss' suggestions where, we believe, the English presently in use by the profession, such as injury for *shang* and generate for *sheng*, does adequately convey the professional Chinese meaning. We have also left in this translation a number of Chinese technical terms which we hope enter the English language TCM vocabulary. In each case, the first few times the Chinese term appears, an English translation is also given.

Bob Flaws
Boulder, CO
March 9, 1992

Translator's Preface
Fu Qing-zhu, His Life & Works

Fu Qing Zhu Nu Ke (Fu Qing-zhu's Gynecology) is indisputably the single most important premodern Chinese text on *fu ke,* a.k.a. *nu ke,* or gynecology. Since it was written in the early Qing Dynasty, it has been one of the most cited of all Chinese *fu ke* books. Many of the most commonly used TCM *fu ke* prescriptions stem from this text as do many of TCM's theories concerning disease mechanism and pattern differentiation *vis a vis* gynecology. Although the number of TCM gynecology texts has steadily increased since Fu Qing-zhu's time and although there are other great names in TCM gynecology, such as Zhang Jing-yue, Ye Tian-shi, and Chen Ze-ming, no TCM *fu ke* specialist can afford to be ignorant of Fu Qing-zhu and his work.

This book originally consisted of 4 books or volumes. We have presented these as Books 1-4. Books 1 and 2 deal with *nu ke* or the general practice of gynecology. Books 3 and 4 deal with *chan hou* or birthing and postpartum disorders. Because *nu ke* or gynecology is the larger field inclusive of birthing and postpartum diseases, there is some overlap in the second two volumes with material presented in the first two. For instance, *beng lou* or profuse uterine bleeding is discussed in Chapter 5, Book 2 under *nu ke* and also in Chapter 2, Book 3 under the heading *chan hou zhu zheng zhi fa* or treatment methods for various postpartum disease. Because of this overlap, the second two books are generally considered supplementary to the first two. As a matter of historical fact, the second two books were added after the first two had been compiled and published long after Fu Qing-zhu's death. (As the reader will see, Books 1 & 2 are written in a different style from 3 & 4.) Although these two parts may, in some cases, discuss similar topics, their contents — case studies, prescriptions, etc.— rarely overlap. Therefore, this second section is nonetheless important.

Two books on medicine are credited to Fu Qing-zhu. These are *Fu Qing Zhu Nu Ke* and *Fu Qing Zhu Nan Ke (Fu Qing-zhu's Men's [Urogenital] Diseases)*. At first, it seems curious that these books by Fu Qing-zhu are so similar in content to the *Bian Zheng Lu (Records on Pattern Discrimination)* and *Shi Shi Mi Lu (The Stone Study Secret Records)* of Chen Shi-duo, the famous early Qing Dynasty physician. These similarities have provoked more than mere curiosity. Chen Shi-duo was one of Fu Qing-zhu's pupils. Although Fu Qing-zhu, the author credited for the present work, died a little more than 300 years ago, the authorship of his works has been the subject of on-going debate for the last three centuries. Some maintain that Chen Shi-duo's works were all actually written by Fu Qing-zhu. If this is true, Chen Shi-duo was little more than a plagiarist. Others assert that Fu Qing-zhu himself did not write anything in his lifetime and that all works attributed to him are simply records of his lectures. These were then edited by Chen Shi-duo and other unknown students of Fu Qing-zhu. Still others hold that Chen Shi-duo was indeed the author of these works and that, at a later date, other of Fu Qing-zhu's pupils extracted from them the parts that they believed to be Fu Qing-zhu's writings and published these as independent works in memory of their teacher. According to this point of view, these are what we now know as *Fu Qing Zhu Nu Ke* and *Fu Qing Zhu Nan Ke.*

Most probably, all these works were written by Chen Shi-duo who named two of them after his teacher as an expression of his gratitude and respect and as a way to accord these works greater significance. By naming these books after the more famous Fu Qing-zhu, this would attract more favorable attention and thus more readers to these books. This has been a common practice throughout the history of Chinese medicine. For instance, the titles of numerous Chinese medical books contain the name of the Yellow Emperor who is but a legendary figure in Chinese history.

The arising of this dispute is also readily understandable. The *Fu Qing Zhu Nu Ke* was not officially published until 1827 when all the works in question had been in circulation anonymously for 150 years or so. Because of this, it is natural that the authorship should have become a mystery. Another fact accounting for this dispute is that, because Fu Qing-zhu is so prominent a figure in the history of Chinese culture, politics, and medicine, things involving him cannot be passed over lightly. In addition, these works, and the *Fu Qing Zhu Nu Ke* in particular, are too important not to be the focus of research in the TCM circle. As the most important medical works of the late Ming and early Qing, they are a precious legacy in TCM.

As is well-known, few outstanding Chinese TCM doctors in history were not also celebrated writers and politicians, and the life of Fu Qing-zhu was particularly a life tinged with heroism and full of undaunted struggle for the freedom of his nation. In fact, his life was so instructive and thrilling, it could easily be the basis for a spell-binding novel.

Fu Qing-zhu (1607-1684) was born in Tai Yuan, Shanxi, into an intellectual family known for its study and practice of medicine. He was a well-educated man infused with wide-ranging interests. Fu was outstanding in literature, poetry, history, calligraphy, painting, Chinese phonetics, the Daoist classics, and Buddhist scripture. As a child, he showed himself to be exceptionally talented. He also had such a remarkable memory that he could recite by heart anything he read but once. At the young age of 14, he passed the imperial examination at the county level and became a doctor-elect (equivalent to *xiu cai*). At 20, he was granted the *lin sheng* or the position of a paid *xiu cai*. This was a privileged position and great honor for which many intellectuals strived their entire lives to gain. At such a young age, Fu Qing-zhu was on the threshold of the yamen and on the border of the ruling class, the class of Confucian officials. In fact, by this time, Fu Qing-zhu had already established close relations with many of the most powerful men of his day. From the point of view of Confucian officialdom, Fu seemed to have bright prospects in store.

However, seeing the corruption and vicious strife amongst the politicians of his day, Fu Qing-zhu turned his back on such a life. Unlike the majority of intellectuals of his time, he regarded fame, personal gain, and power as clouds in the sky, transient and fleeting, which are scattered and gone in the flash of a moment. This did not mean, however, that he adopted a passive attitude towards life. While he cast away without regret the seeming golden opportunity to gain position as a ruling official, he fought vehemently for social justice. In 1636, when he heard that Yuan Ji-xian, an honest and upright governor and friend of his, had been framed by a clique of ministers at court, he defied a distance of more than a 1000 *li* and travelled on foot all the way to the capital in order to free Yuan Ji-xian. After successfully persuading a few influential persons to support him, Fu Qing-zhu knelt before the palace, appealing to the emperor for the rehabilitation of his friend and honest governor. This heroic deed took great courage, determination, and resourcefulness to accomplish, for it well might have incurred imminent danger or even death. At that time, any expression of disagreement with, let alone defiance of a decision, however absurd, made by a superior, to say nothing of the emperor, might be declared a crime.

1664 was an eventful year. It saw the collapse of the Ming Dynasty and, after terrible social tumult, the establishment of a new dynasty which was to last for more than two centuries. During this new dynasty, the Han nationality, the majority of the population in China, suffered a barbarous, bloody oppression by a minority, the Manchu. As a Han and Chinese patriot, Fu felt ashamed at becoming the subject of an alien regime. Therefore, he fled to the mountains. He abandoned his comfortable life and voluntarily chose the life of a secluded hermit, living in a mountain cave in Daoist costume, yellow cap and red robe, in memory of the overthrown dynasty. The rulers of the last dynasty were named Zhu, a homonym of cinnabar or the red color, thus the red robe. Whereas the Han, who are all supposed to be offsprings of the Yellow Emperor, regard highly the yellow color, and thus the yellow cap.

During this time, Fu was in close contact with other patriots who were still fighting against the Manchu. To avoid trouble, he often had to change his name. His original name was Fu Ding-chen. In Chinese, *ding chen* means important minister or, literally, a minister who can support heaven, *i.e.*, the court. Obviously, he could no longer use this name since he no longer supported the current regime. His style or literary name was formerly Green Bamboo (*qing zhu*). This is pronounced the same as the name by which he is presently known. In his resistance work against the foreign regime, Fu cleverly made use of a pun and changed the character *zhu* to give his name a new significance. Instead of *zhu*, bamboo, he wrote the last part of his name *zhu*, to rule or conquer. Since the *qing* for green is a homonym for *qing*, the name of the Manchu dynasty, his new name implied the conquering or ruling of the Manchu. In 1654, Fu Qing-zhu was put into prison on charges of attempting to overthrow the rule of the Manchu, but he was soon after released thanks to the efforts of his friends.

After a period of bloody suppression, the ruling class of the Manchu changed tactics in their effort to consolidate their rule. They put on a smiling face and tried to allure distinguished Han personages to join them in their government as collaborators. Fu Qing-zhu was one of those that the Manchu rulers fastened upon. Thus, he was offered a high position in the court. But Fu Qing-zhu was determined to decline this so-called honor. Because his enemies pressed him so hard to join the ruling clique, he at last pretended to be paralysed. This was an easy job since he was a proficient physician. However, the officials concerned were equally determined. Such an appointment was an imperial decree. It was their job to see, on pain of the emperor's displeasure, that it was executed. Therefore, they decided to carry Fu Qing-zhu to the capital on his bed. When the procession approached the gate of the capital where he was met and saluted by a large party headed by the premier, Fu Qing-zhu refused to return the greeting or to go one step further no matter how hard his escort and the premier tried to persuade him.

Such a refusal could be taken as willful defiance of an imperial decree and Fu Qing-zhu could have faced capital punishment. Fu Qing-zhu was clearly aware of this and was willing to accept this consequence. However, his challenge was not answered. Instead, he was conferred an honorary title and permitted to return home. However, for such a title, Fu Qing-zhu was required to pay tribute and express his gratitude to the emperor in person. In those days, a subject was required to chant, "Thank Your Majesty for Your kindness", either in front of or behind the Son of Heaven whenever one received an imperial edict, even if such an edict was a demotion or order to commit suicide.

However, Fu Qing-zhu was Fu Qing-zhu. He did not care a bit about such etiquette. As a last resort, the premier had to order him carried into court by force. During the imperial audience, Fu stood with his head up, showing no sign of yielding. And, to irritate the emperor on purpose, he refused to kneel down. Kneeling in the emperor's presence was the minimum expression of one's recognition of the emperor's sacred right and grace. Seeing that a tragedy might break out any moment, the premier stepped forward to pull Fu Qing-zhu to kneel. To everyone's unexpected surprise, Fu Qing-zhu then lay down on the ground in a show of mock excessive humility. To cover this intentional farce, the premier hurriedly announced, "All right, all right, he has paid his tribute to Your Majesty." When Fu was leaving the capital, all the court ministers and generals were ordered to give him a special send-off.

While Fu Qing-zhu showed himself to be an undaunted rebel against any form of oppression, he also practiced as a true Daoist or Buddhist, showing laudable kindness, generosity, and warm-heartedness to the lower classes. For most of his life, Fu Qing-zhu practiced medicine and his lofty spirit was most fully demonstrated in his treatment of patients. One day, a scholar who had been living in utter destitution was dying. The last wish he expressed was to know the correct diagnosis of his disease from Fu Qing-zhu. This might seem like an easy wish to realize but, in effect, in those days, it was not. First the dying man feared that he did not have enough money to pay such a famous doctor, and, secondly, he lived hundreds of *li* away from his admired physician. One of his friends walked a couple of days' journey until he found Fu Qing-zhu. The man begged for a diagnosis and prescription alone. Beyond that he expected nothing. To his surprise, no sooner had he finished his request than Fu Qing-zhu got ready and set off on foot to see the dying patient.

Another time, Fu Qing-zhu visited a temple. He was studying some statues when he heard a groan. He asked the monk accompanying him who it was. When he was told that a poor man was lying somewhere in the temple waiting for death, Fu hurriedly rushed to find him. After examining the poor man, he immediately set out to buy the required medicines. The man was saved in the end but the story does not end there. After that, each time Fu Qing-zhu went to the same temple, he met with several more such cases. At last, his suspicion was aroused. After investigation, he found that these cases were a fraud, well designed by the monk whose hands had been greased by some officials. Fu Qing-zhu had previously refused these collaborators as patients, but they were, nonetheless, eager to obtain certain prescriptions from him for their diseases.

It is said that Fu Qing-zhu's house was crowded from morning till night with patients rich or poor from far and near. Of course, these people came to him not merely to make use of his generosity. They came to see Fu Qing-zhu out of confidence in his marvelous technique. Many a difficult case was cured by him and many a long bed-stricken patient was helped up again by Fu Qing-zhu. To accommodate so many patients and to impart his medicine, he set up a school of hygiene. Not a few outstanding physicians in the early years of the Qing Dynasty were trained under him. Even today, the hygiene school he founded is preserved in Taiyuan, Shanxi Province. This may well be the only medical institution so well preserved since the days of imperial China.

Fu Qing-zhu was dubbed by his contemporaries as Divine Doctor, the most sacred acclaim a premodern Chinese physician could enjoy. His attainment in medicine was closely related to his personality. He was a wide reader with a perfect command of the medical classics. This erudition laid a solid foundation for his further probing. But, Fu Qing-zhu was not a person who slavishly followed his predecessors. Through his diligent study, Fu acquired the splendid heritage earlier generations had left, but, starting from that point, he advanced further, leaving us his own valuable legacy. His *Fu Qing Zhu Nu Ke* cannot fail to impress anyone with his profound knowledge, originality, and creativity. For the *Fu Qing Zhu Nu Ke* is not a copy or a collection or notes of works by some earlier authority, as many Chinese medical works were and are. In it, we do not find numerous quotes and citations from earlier classics as is often the case with other premodern texts. Instead, it is full of criticism and the correction of conventional, popular mistakes.

The author, in many places and conspicuously, warns that blind worship of ancient prescriptions is harmful. Quite a number of diagnoses of diseases covered in this book are contrary to those made by Zhang Zhong-jing, for instance. And quite a number of Fu Qing-zhu's formulas cannot be found in any of the earlier classics. Later generations have found that these new diagnoses and fresh discussions on disease mechanisms corrected millennia-old mistakes and that Fu Qing-zhu's prescriptions are more effective than many earlier ones. For example, morning sickness had been assumed to be due to spleen/stomach vacuity. This hypothesis had been supported by a number of medical classics and had easily been taken for granted since it mainly manifests as a series of gastrointestinal complaints. However, based on his keen observation and rich experience, Fu Qing-zhu advanced an opposite, yet correct diagnosis. Morning sickness, Fu says, is caused by the urgency of liver qi. Likewise, *Sheng Hua Tang*, a quite simple formula, is Fu Qing-zhu's creation with which no TCM doctor of today is unacquainted. This is indeed a miraculous formula capable of treating a variety of women's diseases and, so far, no other formula can be used as a substitute in certain cases. Other examples like this are numerous: *Wan Dai Tang, Gu Ben Zhi Beng Tang, Tong Ru Chang Ning Tang,* etc. etc. It is no wonder that Fu Qing-zhu's *Nu Ke* is looked upon as one of the most authoritative works on women's disease in TCM.

Another feature of the book that strikes the reader is its practical value. As the author himself declares, each case study is based on his own experience. Therefore, each of his prescriptions is time-honored. Besides, the language is terse without complicated theoretical exposition. In particular, Fu Qing-zhu's writing style deserves mention. He used a purely colloquial language that was probably understandable by an illiterate of his times. This is, perhaps, the most convincing evidence that his works were, in fact, a compilation of his lectures. The original editor(s), most likely his pupils, preserved this conversational tone and style on purpose as a sign of respect for their master. This merits all the more compliment in view of the fact that most premodern Chinese scholars made a fetish of a highly literary style. The fact that Fu Qing-zhu's style is easy for us to read today is also accounted for, in part, by the fact that Fu Qing-zhu lived in an age not too distant from our own.

We translators wish to thank Blue Poppy Press for entrusting such a book to our care and ministrations. The editors of this press must have a good eye for and be very proficient in TCM, since even for a senior Chinese TCM doctor, it is not easy to pick those books most worth translating from the enormous wealth of Chinese TCM literature. The editors of Blue Poppy Press, in commissioning this translation, no doubt believe that it will benefit women in the Western world. If one of the translator's experiences is any proof of that, we also believe this will be true. In 1989, one of the translators was acting as an interpreter for a delegation from Minnesota. A female member of that delegation had long suffered from a certain gynecologic disease and her condition was deteriorating because of her heavy schedule. The translator recommended to her to try seeing a TCM doctor. A single dose and her problems were alleviated! This woman expressed her wonder, saying that she had seen various doctors for years. Nonetheless, her condition had gotten steadily worse to the point that she had previously lost all hope of recovery. What prescription worked so miraculously? It was one of those from *Fu Qing Zhu Nu Ke.*

Acknowledgements

Thanks are due to Dr. Dong Huang-jun and Mrs. Xie Guanghua who never failed to give the translators enlightening explanation on many TCM technical problems whenever they were consulted and whose profound learning has struck the translators deeply. Thanks must also go to Mr. Dong Yi-lun who readily wrote the Chinese title of this book in a very beautiful calligraphy. The translators are also much indebted to Mr. Meng Jian and Mr. Yu Zhong-wen who helped solve many problems concerning the typing of this manuscript.

Yang Shou-zhong
North China Coalmines Medical College
Tangshan, Hebei, PRC

Table of Contents

Editor's Preface v

Translator's Preface xi

Book 1: *Nu Ke*/Gynecology

Chapter 1: *Dai Xia*/Abnormal Vaginal Discharge 3
- White Vaginal Discharge 3
- Green-blue Vaginal Discharge 6
- Yellow Vaginal Discharge 8
- Black Vaginal Discharge 10
- Red Vaginal Discharge 12

Chapter 2: *Xue Beng*/Profuse Uterine Bleeding 17
- Profuse Bleeding with Dimness & Darkness 17
- Profuse Bleeding in Old Women 19
- Profuse Bleeding in Young Women 21
- (Sexual) Union Causing Bleeding 22
- Depression Knotting Profuse Bleeding 24
- Profuse Bleeding Due to Wrenching & Falling 26
- Profuse Bleeding Due to Great Heat in the Sea of Blood 28

Chapter 3: *Tiao Jing*/Balancing the Menses 31
- Menstruation Ahead of Schedule 31
- Menstruation Behind Schedule 33
- Menstruation Early, Late, At No Fixed Intervals 35
- Menstruation Comes Once Every Several Months 37
- Recurrent Menstruation in Old Women 38

Menstruation Suddenly Comes, Suddenly Ceases, Sometimes Pain, Sometimes Stops 40
Menstruation Not Yet Arrived Preceded by Abdominal Ache 42
Menstruation Followed by Lower Abdominal Aching & Pain 43
Abdominal Aching & Vomiting of Blood Preceding Menstruation 45
Aching & Pain Below the Umbilicus Before the Period is About to Come 47
Excessive Menstruation 49
Watery Discharge Before Menstruation 51
Hemafecia Prior to Menstruation 52
Premature Menopause 55

Book 2: *Nu Ke*/Gynecology (Continued)

Chapter 1: ***Ren Shen*****/Pregnancy** 61
Pregnancy Malign Blockage (*i.e.*, Morning Sickness 61
Swelling & Edema in Pregnancy 63
Lower Abdominal Pain in Pregnancy 66
Dry Mouth & Sore Throat in Pregnancy 67
Vomiting, Diarrhea, & Abdominal Pain in Pregnancy 69
Fetal Suspension with Lateral Costal Pain in Pregnancy 71
Impact Injury in Pregnancy 73
Hematuria in Pregnancy, (also) Called Fetal Leakage 75
Fetal Crying in Pregnancy 77
Fetal Mania, (*i.e.*), Lumbar & Abdominal Pain, Thirst, Sweating, & Mania in Pregnancy 78
Falling Fetus (Due to) Excessive Anger During Pregnancy 80

Chapter 2: *Xiao Chan*/Small Birth, (*i.e.*, Miscarriage) 83
Miscarriage (Due to) Sexual Intercourse 83
Miscarriage (Due to) Wrenching & Contusion 85
Miscarriage with Dry, Knotted Stools 86
Aversion to Cold & Abdominal Pain with Miscarriage 88
Miscarriage (Due to) Great Anger 90

Chapter 3: *Nan Chan*/Difficult Delivery 93
Blood Vacuity Difficult Delivery 93
Difficult Delivery (Due to) the Joined Bones Not Opening 95
Hand or Foot Comes Down First Difficult Delivery, (*i.e.*, Breach Presentation) 97
Qi Counterflow Difficult Delivery 99
Child Dead at the Birth Gate Difficult Delivery 101
Dead Child Within the Abdomen Difficult Delivery 102

Chapter 4: *Zheng Chan*/Normal Delivery 105
Normal Delivery (but) the Placenta Does Not Descend 105
Normal Delivery (but) Qi Vacuity, Blood Dizziness 109
Normal Delivery (but) Blood Dizziness (&) Loss of Speech 111
Normal Delivery (but) Vanquished Blood Attacks the Heart (Causing) Dizziness (&) Mania 112
Normal Delivery (but) Intestinal Prolapse 114

Chapter 5: *Chan Hou*/Postpartum (Disorders) 117
Postpartum Lower Abdominal Pain 117
Postpartum Asthma 120
Postpartum Aversion to Cold (&) Body Shivering 122

Postpartum Nausea, Retching (&) Vomiting 123
Postpartum Profuse (Uterine) Bleeding 125
Postpartum Incessant Dribbling (of Blood Due to) the *Bao Tai* Being Injured by Hand 127
Postpartum Swelling (&) Edema of the Four Limbs 129
Postpartum Exit of Fleshy Fiber 131
Postpartum Liver Atony 132
Postpartum Qi (&) Blood Dual Vacuity Breast Milk Not Descending 134
Postpartum Depression (&) Knotting Breast Mild Not Flowing Freely 135

Book 3: *Chan Hou*/Birthing & Afterwards

Chapter 1: *Chan Hou Zong Lun*/An Overview of Postpartum (Disorders) 141

Chapter 2: *Chan Qian Hou Fang Zheng Yi Ji*/Indications (&) Contraindications of Pre (&) Postpartum Disorders 147

Normal Delivery 147
Injured Delivery 147
Balancing (or Regulating) Delivery 148
Hastening Birth 149
Frozen Delivery 149
Hot Delivery 149
Transverse Delivery 150
Placenta Intestine Delivery (*i.e.*, Wound Umbilical Cord Delivery) 151
Difficult Delivery 151
Dead (Fetus) Delivery 152
Descending the Fetal (Placenta) 152
Severing the Navel (*i.e.*, the Umbilical Cord) 154
Treatment Methods for the Newly Birthed 157
Ten Mistakes in Using Medicinals Postpartum 158

Postpartum Cold (&) Heat 159
Before Birth Contraction of Cold Injury, Epidemic Disease, Malaria, Miscarriage, etc. 161

Chapter 3: ***Chan Hou Zhu Zheng Zhi Fa*/Treatment Methods for Various Postpartum Conditions** 163
Blood Clots 163
Blood Dizziness 166
Inversion Condition 171
Profuse (Uterine) Bleeding 174
Shortness of Breath Similar to Asthma 177
Confused Speech, Confused Vision 179
Food Injury 182
Indignation (&) Anger 184
Quasi-Malaria 186
Quasi-Cold Injury Conditions of the Two Yang 189
Quasi-Cold Injury Conditions of the Three Yin 191
Quasi-Windstroke 194
Quasi-Tetany 197
Sweating 198
Thief (*i.e.*, Night) Sweating 201
Thirsty Mouth (with) Simultaneous Inhibited Urination 202
Enuresis 203

Book 4: *Chan Hou*/Birthing & Afterwards (Continued)

***Chan Hou*/Birthing & Afterwards** 207
Mistaken Damage of the Urinary Bladder 207
Contraction of Strangury 208
Frequent Urination 209
Diarrhea 210
Whole Grains Not Transformed (*i.e.*, Undigested Food in the Stools) 213

Dysentery 215
Sudden Chaos (*i.e.*, Choleric Diseases) 219
Counterflow Retching (&) Inability to Eat 221
Coughing 223
Water Swelling 226
Flowing, Pouring (Sore) 228
Inflation (&) Distention 230
Racing Heart (&) Fright Palpitations 233
Steaming Bone 235
Heart Pain 237
Abdominal Pain 238
Lower Abdominal Pain 239
Vacuity Taxation 240
Generalized Body Aching (&) Pain 240
Lumbar Pain 241
Lateral Costal Pain 243
Genital Pain 244
The Lochia 246
Mammary *Yong* 248
Severe Wind 251
Aphasia 251

Bu Bian/Appendix 253
Postpartum Constipation 253
Treating Postpartum Chicken Claw Wind 254
Treating Generalized Water Swelling 255

Index 257

Book 1

Nu Ke
Gynecology

Chapter 1

Dai Xia
Abnormal Vaginal Discharge

All types of *dai xia* or abnormal vaginal discharge are dampness patterns. The reason it is called *dai* is that it is due to failure of the *dai mai* or girdle vessel to astringe.[1] As long as it has free and open access to the *ren* (conception) and *du* (governing) vessels, the *dai mai* is not diseased unless the *ren* and *du mai* are diseased. When the *dai mai,* which is the vessel that astringes the ligation of the *bao tai* or uterus-fetus [2], is feeble, it finds it difficult to uplift the ligation and the *bao tai* becomes *bu gu* or unconsolidated. It is said, therefore, that a weak *dai mai* leads to the fetus easily dropping and that injury to the girdle vessel renders the fetus insecure. The *dai mai* may be damaged not only by wrenching and contusion but also by overindulgence in sexual intercourse or wanton drinking. These may not cause the suffering of aching and pain but can

---

1 In Chinese, *dai* means belt or girdle. *Xia* means downward. However, as a compound term, *dai xia* means abnormal vaginal discharge. This name refers to both this disease's occurring below the belt and also to its being seen as largely a dysfunction of the *dai mai* or girdle vessel.

2 This is a very difficult term to translate. *Bao* refers to the *bao gong* or uterus. *Tai* most often means fetus but can refer to the placenta. Sometimes this term refers to the uterus, sometimes to the fetus, and sometimes to both.

cause the harm of insidious exhaustion. As a result, the qi is not able to transform the *jing shui* or menstrual flow[3] and this then is the cause of *dai bing* or vaginal discharge disease. Because of this, *dai xia* is common in nuns, widows, and married women but rarely seen in maidens. Furthermore, how can such a problem not be brewed if, in addition, spleen qi is vacuous, liver qi is depressed, damp qi has invaded, or hot qi is oppressing?

(Some) women, therefore, may suffer all year round from constant running without check from the lower orifice of a whitish fluid which is like snivel and saliva and which, in a serious cases, may have an offensively foul odor. This is called *bai dai* or white vaginal discharge. Such *bai dai* points to exuberant dampness with debilitated fire and a depressed liver with weak qi. This leads to damage and injury of spleen/earth with the qi of damp earth falling downward. As a result, spleen essence, no longer able to bear its responsibility (of keeping to its abode), fails to transform the *ying*[4] and blood into the *jing* shui or menstruate. Rather, it turns into something whitish and slippery which pours out from the secret gate beyond control.

The appropriate treatment method is to greatly supplement spleen and stomach qi and aided by the introduction of liver-soothing medicinals. When wind/wood is no longer

---

3 *Jing* means channel or canal. It also refers to *yue jing* or moon flow, *i.e.*, menstruation. *Shui* means water. As a compound term, *jing shui* is used when an author wishes to underscore the yin fluid aspect of the menstruate.

4 *Ying* refers to the constructive qi as opposed to the *wei* or defensive qi.

blocked in the earth[5], earth qi may rise to heaven[6] above by itself. And when spleen qi is fortified, damp qi is dispersed. Thus, automatically, there is no further trouble from white vaginal discharge. The formula to use is ***Wan Dai Tang*** (End Discharge Decoction):

Rhizoma Atractylodis Macrocephalae (*Bai Zhu*), 1 *liang*, stir-fried with earth
Radix Dioscoreae Oppositae (*Shan Yao*), 1 *liang*, stir-fried
Radix Panacis Ginseng (*Ren Shen*), 2 *qian*
Radix Albus Paeoniae Lactiflorae (*Bai Shao*), 5 *qian*, stir-fried with wine
Semen Plantaginis (*Che Qian Zi*), 3 *qian*, stir-fried with wine
Rhizoma Atractylodis (*Cang Zhu*), 3 *qian*, processed
Radix Glycyrrhizae (*Gan Cao*), 1 *qian*
Pericarpium Citri Reticulatae (*Chen Pi*), 5 *fen*
Herba Seu Flos Carbonisatus Schizonepetae Tenuifoliae (*Hei Jie Sui*) 5 *fen*
Radix Bupleuri (*Chai Hu*), 6 *fen*

Decoct in water and take. Two *ji* (literally formula, but it means a packet of medicinals) will effect mitigation; 4 *ji* will stop (the discharge); and 6 *ji* will effect complete recovery from *bai dai*. This formula is a method to treat simultaneously the three channels of the spleen, stomach, and the liver. It is able to supplement by way of dissipating and to disperse through upbearing. When liver/wood qi is opened and raised, liver blood is no longer dry. Then how can it descend to restrain spleen/earth? When the source of spleen/earth is supplemented and boosted, spleen qi is no longer damp. Then how can it be

---

5 Here, the word earth refers to both the lower part of the body and the spleen/stomach.

6 Heaven in this case refers to the upper part of the body.

difficult to separate and disperse water qi? As to the reason for supplementing the stomach together with the spleen, the external is reached from the internal. Unless stomach qi is made strong, the spleen cannot turn from weak to effulgent. In this sense, supplementing the stomach is as good as supplementing the spleen.

Qing Dai
Green-blue Vaginal Discharge

(Some) women have vaginal discharge of a green-blue color or, in serious cases, a green color like mung beans which is sticky and runs constantly with a fishy smell. This is called *qing dai* or greenish blue vaginal discharge. It is (due to) damp heat of the liver channel. Since the liver pertains to wood which is green-blue in color, vaginal discharge running like mung bean juice is obviously a disease ascribed to liver/wood. Liver/wood likes to be moistened by water above all, and dampness is an accumulation of water. It would seem, therefore, that dampness is not among that which is hated by the liver/wood. Then how can the pattern of *qing dai* develop? It should be understood that dampness is indeed hated by liver/wood although it favors water, for dampness is the qi of earth. Suppose what is hated is mixed with what is liked. (In such a case,) there would certainly be contravention. Once the nature of the liver is contravened, its qi is sure to counterflow. This qi is inclined to ascend, while dampness tends to descend. Drawn towards each other, these two must stop somewhere in the middle burner, penetrating the *dai mai,* and then are excreted from the secret organ. The reason that the discharge is green-blue or green is none other than that it is transmuted by the qi that is overwhelming liver/wood. If the counterflow is slight, heat is also slight and the color must be green-blue. If the counterflow is serious, heat must be serious and the color must be green. It might seem, therefore, that a green-blue (discharge) is easier to cure than a green (discharge), but, in fact, neither is difficult to treat. Resolving fire within liver/wood and disinhibiting water in the urinary bladder will eliminate the vaginal discharge whether green- blue or green. The formula to use is ***Jia Jian Xiao Yao San*** (Modified Rambling Powder):

Sclerotium Poriae Cocoris (*Fu Ling*), 5 *qian*
Radix Albus Paeoniae Lactiflorae (*Bai Shao*), stir-fried with wine, 5 *qian*
Radix Glycyrrhizae (*Gan Cao*), use raw, 5 *qian*
Radix Bupleuri (*Chai Hu*), 1 *qian*
Herba Artemesiae Capillaris (*Yin Chen*), 3 *qian*
Pericarpium Citri Reticulatae (*Chen Pi*), 1 *qian*
Fructus Gardeniae Jasminoidis (*Zhi Zi*), 3 *qian*, stir-fried

Decoct in water and take. Two *ji* will make (the color) lighter and 4 *ji* will exterminate vaginal discharge, either green-blue or green. More doses are unnecessary. *Xiao Yao San* is composed of medicinals to resolve liver depression. Then why does it treat green-blue vaginal discharge so magically? It is because of the depression of liver qi that damp heat lingers in the liver channel. (Further,) depression invariably results in counterflow and *Xiao Yao San* is (the formula) most capable of resolving the depression and counterflow of the liver. When depressed and counterflow qi is resolved, damp heat will find it difficult to persist. What's more, (because of) dampness-disinhibiting Herba Artemesiae Capillaris and heat-clearing Fructus Gardeniae Jasominoidis, liver qi is cleared. Then, from where can green-blue or green vaginal discharge come by itself? This accounts for the miraculous effectiveness and quick results of this formula. If green-blue vaginal discharge is treated merely by disinhibiting dampness and clearing heat without consideration of liver qi, it can never be stopped.

Huang Dai
Yellow Vaginal Discharge

(Some) women have a yellow colored *dai xia* like strong brown tea with a fishy smell. This is called *huang dai* or yellow vaginal discharge. It is (due to) damp heat of the *ren mai* or conception vessel. Since the *ren mai* does not hold water by nature, how can damp qi enter it to transform into yellow vaginal discharge? It should be understood that the *dai mai* arises transversely and connects freely with the *ren mai*. Whereas the *ren mai* runs straight up and penetrates the lips and teeth, between which there exists an eternal spring that flows down, penetrating the conception vessel to transform into *jing* essence. For that reason, hot qi is kept from surrounding the conception vessel so that the fluids within the mouth can all transform into essence and enter the kidneys. But when hot evils exist in the precincts of the lower burner, fluids are no longer able to transform into essence but transform (instead) into dampness. Dampness, the qi of earth, is, practically (speaking), the intrusion of water. While heat, the qi of fire, is, practically (speaking), generated by wood. Water is black in color and fire is red. When dampness is combined with heat, its transformation into red is made impossible and so is its reinstatement to black. It is boiled down to a sap, (thus) turning yellow. This is a deviation from fire/water transformation to dampness transformation. Nowadays, some people, based on the hypothesis that yellow vaginal discharge is (caused by) damp heat of the spleen, attempt in vain to cure it by means of merely treating the spleen. Their failure results from ignorance of (the fact) that the yellow is transmuted by the cinnabar and origin evils[7] which are synthesized from true fire and true water surrounding the *ren mai* and *bao tai*. How

---

7 *Zhu* or cinnabar implies red or fire. *Yuan* or origin implies black or water.

can it be cured by merely attending to the spleen? The appropriate method is to supplement conception vessel vacuity and to clear flaming kidney fire. Thus success is not far off. The formula to use is ***Yi Huang Tang*** (Change Yellow Decoction):

Radix Dioscoreae Oppositae (*Shan Yao*), stir-fried, 1 *liang*
Semen Euryalis Ferocis (*Qian Shi*), stir-fried, 1 *liang*
Cortex Phellodendri (*Huang Bai*), 2 *qian*, stir-fried with salt water
Semen Plantaginis (*Che Qian Zi*), 1 *qian*, stir-fried with wine
Semen Gingkonis Bilobae (*Bai Guo*), 10 pieces, smashed

Decoct in water. (If) 4 *ji* are taken in succession, complete cure is effected without fail. This formula is able to treat not only *huang dai* but also any other type of vaginal discharge disease. Only it proves still more magical in treating yellow vaginal discharge. Radix Dioscoreae Oppositae and Semen Euryalis Ferocis specifically supplement vacuity of the *ren mai* and are also able to disinhibit water. (Whereas,) the introduction of Semen Gingkonis Bilobae (is able to) lead (these two) into the conception vessel, (thus) providing a short cut. Therefore, the effect is very quick. The reason for using Cortex Phellodendri to clear kidney fire is that as the kidney communicates with and helps the conception vessel. (Therefore,) resolving fire in the kidneys is as good as resolving heat in the *ren mai*.

[Most patterns of vaginal discharge are (due to) spleen dampness. During the initial stage without heat, the disease can be cured for sure by merely supplementing spleen/earth and simultaneously regulating the qi of the *chong* and *ren*. If dampness has persisted for a long time and heat has already been generated, dampness cannot be provided a way out unless kidney fire is cleared. The inclusion of Cortex Phellodendri and Semen Plantaginis in this formula is, (therefore,) admirable.

Radix Dioscoreae Oppositae and Semen Euryalis Ferocis are particularly capable of clearing heat and generating fluids][8]

Hei Dai
Black Vaginal Discharge

(Some) women have a black colored vaginal discharge which, in serious cases, may even be as (black as) black soybean juice with a fishy smell. This is called *hei dai* or black vaginal discharge. It is (due to) extreme fire heat. It may be asked how fire can turn black since it is red in color. It is argued that (black) may be seen only (in case of) extreme cold in the lower (burner). It should be understood that extreme fire can appear, (however,) like water, which is (then) a false appearance. This pattern without exception manifests with abdominal pain, cutting pain on urination, swelling in the secret gate (*i.e.*, the vagina), a red facial complexion or, in chronic cases, leanness with a yellow complexion, food intake double that of normal people, and thirst with hotness in the mouth which can be relieved a little only by drinking cold water. This is excessively effulgent stomach fire which combines with the fires in the life gate[9], urinary bladder, and triple burner which (then) simmer and boil. As boiling ends in drying, (the liquids) are changed into a charcoal color. This is undoubtedly the transmutation of

---

8 The sections in brackets have all been inserted by some later editor.

9 *Ming men* refers to the life gate fire associated with kidney yang or prenatal yang. This fire is the source of all warmth in the body. However, this fire *xiang sheng* or mutually arises with the warmth or fire of the other organs. Therefore, heat in the stomach may cause the *ming men* to flare up in mutual arising.)

extreme fire rather than that of rarely seen cold qi. Such a pattern does not go so far as to develop madness[10] simply by the strength of (still) healthy kidney/water and lung/metal whose life-sustaining and ever-working qi aid in rescuing by moistening the heart and supporting the stomach. When (such) a black vaginal discharge develops, it is always because of fire gathering in the lower (part of the body). Whereas, in the upper, fire never burns. The treatment method is to exclusively apply drainage of fire as the key. Once fire heat retreats, dampness will depart of itself. The formula to use is ***Li Huo Tang*** (Disinhibit Fire Decoction):

Radix Et Rhizoma Rhei (*Da Huang*), 3 *qian*
Rhizoma Atractylodis Macrocephalae (*Bai Zhu*), 5 *qian*, stir-fried
Sclerotium Poriae Cocoris (*Fu Ling*), 3 *qian*
Semen Plantaginis (*Che Qian Zi*), 3 *qian*, stir-fried with wine
Semen Vaccariae Segetalis (*Wang Bu Liu Xing*), 3 *qian*
Rhizoma Coptidis Chinensis (*Huang Lian*), 3 *qian*
Fructus Gardeniae Jasminoidis (*Zhi Zi*), stir-fried, 3 *qian*
Rhizoma Anemarrhenae (*Zhi Mu*), 2 *qian*
Gypsum (*Shi Gao*), 5 *qian*, calcined
Herba Artemesiae Anomalae (*Liu Ji Nu*), 3 *qian*

Decoct in water and take. One *ji* will relieve pain in and disinhibit urination; a second *ji* will change the discharge from black to white; a third *ji* will reduce the white vaginal discharge; 3 more *ji* will effect a complete cure. Some may protest that this formula is too drastic and swift (in action). It should be understood that when fire is raging, there is no alternative method to follow. This is likened to putting down a devastating fire. Given any delay, it will spread and not stop till everything is burned up. The combined use of Radix Et

10 Classically, stomach fire is seen as one of the main causes of madness in Chinese medicine.

Rhizoma Rhei with Rhizoma Coptidis Chinensis, Gypsum, Fructus Gardeniae Jasminoidis, and Rhizoma Anemarrhenae, all of which are cold, cool ingredients, can implement such a swift sweeping. In addition, they are aided by Semen Vaccariae Segetalis and Herba Artemesiae Anomalae which disinhibit dampness in a very radical way. Thus, no chance is left for either dampness or heat to persist. Because Rhizoma Atractylodis Macrocephalae is introduced as an assistant to succor earth, Sclerotium Poriae Cocoris to percolate dampness, and Semen Plantaginis to disinhibit water, fire has to retreat and water is advanced. Thus a *ji ji* diagram forms.[11]

[After recuperation, an abstemious diet should be kept, acrid and heat-generating foods are prohibited, and spleen/earth should be regulated and nurtured. If one, in possession of this formula, takes it whenever one has a relapse, one will unavoidably damage one's *yuan* or original qi. (Therefore,) be cautious!]

Chi Dai
Red Vaginal Discharge

(Some) women may have a red colored vaginal discharge which looks like blood and dribbles continually. This is called *chi dai* or red vaginal discharge. It is, likewise, a damp disease. Dampness is the qi of earth and is, (therefore,) expected to appear whitish yellow. In this case, it is not whitish yellow but

---

11 This refers to the 64 *gua* or hexagrams of the *Yi Jing* or *Classic of Change*. Specifically, the *ji ji* diagram refers to the fourth diagram in the *Kan* Water Palace. This symbolizes water over fire or yin over yang. Since yin naturally moves down and yang naturally moves up, yin and yang or water and fire mutually interpenetrate and mutually transform and promote each other. This diagram is, therefore, a symbol of the mutual harmony and mutual assistance of the correct relationship between fire and water.

red. This is because of fire heat. Fire is red in color; therefore, the discharge is red too. Since the *dai mai* ties to the lower back and the navel near the precincts of consummate yin, there ought be no fire in it. Nonetheless, in this case, a fire pattern appears. Is this because its course leads to the *ming men* or life gate and its fire comes out and burns? It should be understood that the *dai mai* has access or connects freely to the kidneys and kidney qi has access to the liver. When a woman's spleen is injured by worry and (over)thinking and if, in addition, her liver is injured by depression and anger, depressive fire will flame in the liver channel and descend to restrain or overcontrol spleen/earth. (In that case,) because spleen/earth is no longer able to transport and transform, the qi of damp heat is brewed in the *dai mai*. What's more, as it cannot be stored by the liver, blood, too, percolates into the girdle vessel. Because of injured spleen qi which has no strength left to transport and transform, the qi of damp heat, which follows (the damaged spleen) qi, falls and comes out together with blood. (Thus) it exhibits an appearance of something like blood in color. As a matter of fact, blood and dampness are inseparable. People nowadays attribute red vaginal discharge to heart fire. (But) this is wrong. The treatment method must be to clear liver fire and support spleen qi. Thus a cure can be expected soon. The formula to use is ***Qing Gan Zhi Lin Tang*** (Clear the Liver, Stop Dribbling Decoction):

Radix Albus Paeoniae Lactiflorae (*Bai Shao*), 1 *liang*, stir-fried with vinegar
Radix Angelicae Sinensis (*Dang Gui*), 1 *liang*, stir-fried with wine
Radix Rehmanniae (*Sheng Di*), 5 *qian*, stir-fried with wine
Gelatinum Corii Asini (*E Jiao*), 3 *qian*, stir-fried with wheat flour
Cortex Radicis Moutan (*Fen Dan Pi*), 3 *qian*
Cortex Phellodendri (*Huang Bai*), 2 *qian*

Radix Achyranthis Bidentatae (*Niu Xi*), 2 *qian*
Rhizoma Cyperi Rotundi (*Xiang Fu*), 1 *qian*, stir-fried with wine
Fructus Zizyphi Jujubae (*Hong Zao*), 10 pieces
Small black beans (*Xiao Hei Dou*), 1 *liang*

Decoct in water and take. One *ji* will effect mitigation to some degree; a second *ji* will effect mitigation to a greater extent; a fourth *ji* will effect a complete cure; (and) a tenth *ji* will prevent relapse. This formula is designed to solely supplement the blood of the liver without disinhibiting dampness of the spleen at all. This is because the cause of *chi dai* or red vaginal discharge is serious fire with (only) slight dampness. Since the cause of effulgent fire is debilitated blood, supplementation of blood is, (therefore,) sufficient to overcome fire. What's more, because *chi dai* disease results from a combination of water and blood in such a way that dampness in it is hardly identifiable, dampness (must) have entirely transformed into blood too. For that reason, treating the blood also eliminates (this) dampness. Therefore, why take the trouble of specifically disinhibiting dampness? The subtlety of this formula lies in its purely treating the blood with the help of only a small amount of medicinals to clear fire. This accounts for its singular, miraculous effectiveness. Suppose dampness were to be disinhibited, fire would be undesirably conducted down (together with it, thus) rendering it difficult to achieve quick effect. It may be asked, "Sir, you have previously explained (the necessity) of assisting the qi of spleen/earth, but now why (do you recommend) mere supplementation of the blood of liver/wood?" It should be understood that when Radix Albus Paeoniae

Lactiflorae is introduced to level the liver[12], liver qi is (automatically) soothed. (Thus) soothed, liver qi will certainly not restrain or overcontrol spleen/earth. Once the spleen is freed from restraint, spleen/earth naturally becomes effulgent. In this sense, to level the liver is as good as supporting the spleen. Therefore, why include such medicinals as Radix Panacis Ginseng (*Ren Shen*) and Rhizoma Atractylodis Macrocephalae (*Bai Zhu*) only to add trouble?

---

12 *Ping* means to level but it also implies something that is calm. For instance, the Pacific Ocean is called the *Da Ping Hai*, the great level, *i.e.*, pacific, sea. Therefore, *ping gan* means to level the liver as well as to calm the liver. When it is used to describe the restraint of arrogantly ascending liver yang, the sense of levelling takes on a clearly spatial implication. Here, *ping gan* implies that liver qi, when it becomes stagnant and accumulates, rises up from the lower to the middle burners to overcontrol and attack the spleen. It should be remembered that Radix Albus Paeoniae Lactiflorae has an astringing and restraining function on the yang. Thus *ping gan* has a somewhat larger meaning than simply *he gan* or harmonizing the liver or *shu gan*, soothing the liver.

Chapter 2

Xue Beng
Profuse Uterine Bleeding

Xue Beng Hun An
Profuse Bleeding with Dimness & Darkness

(In some) women with sudden profuse (uterine) bleeding, both eyes become black and dark. There is dimness (of vision) and dizziness with sudden collapse and loss of consciousness of human affairs. People all declare this to be (due to) blood stirred by exuberant fire. This fire, however, is not replete fire but vacuity fire. Physicians tend to employ (blood)-stopping and astringing ingredients whenever they meet (a case of) *xue beng* or profuse (uterine) bleeding, and they may indeed achieve some temporary effects (thereby). But, if one does not use yin-supplementing medicinals, this makes it easy for vacuity fire to surge and attack. Thus, it is quite likely for relapse to follow in the wake of stopping (bleeding, *i.e., zhi xue* therapy) with some cases even not being able to be cured entirely for years. Hence, it follows that stop-flooding medicinals should never be used alone and that it is necessary to stop flooding through the method of supplementing yin. The formula to use is *Gu Ben Zhi Beng Tang* (Consolidate the Root, Stop Flooding Decoction):

Radix Coquitus Rehmanniae (*Da Shu Di*), 1 *liang*, steamed nine times
Rhizoma Atractylodis Macrocephalae (*Bai Zhu*), 1 *liang*, char-fried with earth
Radix Astragali Seu Hedysari (*Huang Qi*), 3 *qian*, use fresh
Radix Angelicae Sinensis (*Dang Gui*), 5 *qian*, washed with wine
Rhizoma Carbonisata Zingiberis (*Hei Jiang*), 2 *qian*
Radix Panacis Ginseng (*Ren Shen*), 3 *qian*

Decoct in water and take. One *ji* will stem uterine bleeding and 10 *ji* will prevent relapse. If the ingredients are reduced to half their amounts for fear of this formula being too heavy, then its strength would become too weak to stem the bleeding. The subtlety of this formula lies in its supplementing the blood without taking the trouble to stop it at all and its not supplementing so much the blood as the qi, nor supplementing so much the qi as fire. If profuse uterine bleeding is so serious as to cause dark eyes, clouding, and dizziness, blood has already run out and what is left is but a thread of qi to provide protection and (attempt to) sustain (life). If qi is not immediately supplemented to generate the blood but, instead, supplementation of blood takes precedence at the neglect of qi, then tangible blood can hardly be generated quickly (enough) while intangible qi would be sure to disperse to nothing. That is why qi is first supplemented instead of blood. If, however, qi alone is supplemented, blood will not be generated easily, and, if blood alone is supplemented to the exclusion of fire, blood will certainly become stagnant and, (therefore,) cannot be generated quickly by the qi. Furthermore, Rhizoma Carbonisata Zingiberis, which can conduct the blood back within the channels, has the admirable effect of astringing at the same time as it supplements. Thus, it is used together with qi and blood supplementing medicinals.

[In case of several day old, profuse uterine bleeding with several *dou* of blood shed, all six pulses[1] may become absent and only a faint breath is left in the nose. In this case, do not administer this formula impetuously for fear that the qi, which is about to desert, may not be able to endure such strong supplementation. For the strong case, administer 3 *qian* of steamed Radix Panacis Ginseng (*Liao Ren Shen*) which is decocted and taken with one *qian* of charred, powdered Rhizoma Guanzhong (*Guan Zhong*). Then, after the breath becomes a little stronger, administer the (above) formula, still with one *qian* of charred, powdered Rhizoma Guanzhong brewed along with it. This (prescription) is effective without fail. For the weak case, administer three *qian* of charred, powdered Rhizoma Guanzhong brewed in good quality Shaoxing wine. Do not administer the above formula until breath has become smooth and the spirit clear. Radix Codonopsis Pilosulae (*Dang Shen*) can be substituted for Radix Panacis Ginseng. (In that case,) take the decoction still with one *qian* of charred, powdered Rhizoma Guanzhong brewed along with it.]

Lao Nian Xue Beng
Profuse Bleeding in Old Women

Older women with profuse uterine bleeding can also have the same condition of clouding and darkening of the eyes similar to *xue beng hun an* above. People suppose (this is due to) the vacuity (common) to the elderly. Who would suspect the cause to be indiscreet sexual intercourse? The formula to use is *Jia*

1 This refers to the *cun kou* pulses of the radial arteries at the styloid processes of the wrists. These are divided into *cun, guan,* and *chi* positions on the two wrists which altogether make six pulse positions.

Jian Dang Gui Bu Xue Tang (Modified *Dang Gui*, Supplement the Blood Decoction):

Radix Angelicae Sinensis (*Dang Gui*), 1 *liang*, washed with wine
Radix Astragali Seu Hedysari (*Huang Qi*), 1 *liang*, use raw
Radix Pseudoginseng (*San Qi*), powdered root, 3 *qian*
Folium Mori Albi (*Sang Ye*), 14 leaves

Decoct in water and take. Two *ji* (and) bleeding is stopped a little; 4 *ji* prevent relapse. It is necessary, however, to abstain from sexual desire to root out (the cause of) this disease. If one surrenders to sexual desire, serious relapse will inevitably arise. (*Dang Gui) Bu Xue Tang* is a divine formula capable of supplementing both qi and blood. Radix Pseudoginseng is a wonder--working drug for stopping bleeding. Together with Folium Mori Albi, it has the admirable effect of not only enriching kidney yin but astringing (blood). However, because old women are depleted of yin essence, this formula can only be used to stem the leakage for the time being. Although it is indeed magically effective, an ever-lasting effect cannot be expected from it. (This is because) the medicinals to supplement essence are not sufficient in it. After 4 *ji* are taken, the following should be added:

Rhizoma Atractylodis Macrocephalae (*Bai Zhu*), 5 *qian*
Radix Coquitus Rehmanniae (*Shu Di*), 1 *liang*
Radix Dioscoreae Oppositae (*Shan Yao*), 4 *qian*
Tuber Ophiopogonis Japonicae (*Mai Dong*), 3 *qian*
Fructus Schizandrae Chinensis (*Bei Wu Wei*), 1 *qian*

Take 100 *ji* and *beng lou* (literally flooding and leakage but usually translated as uterine bleeding) will be rooted out.

[Profuse uterine bleeding can also be met with in old widows. (In this case,) it must be caused by qi surging into the blood chamber. Add to the (above) formula 3 *qian* of charred Radix Albus Paeoniae Lactiflorae (*Hang Shao*) and 3 *qian* of charred Rhizoma Guanzhong (*Guan Zhong*). This is extremely efficacious.]

Shao Fu Xue Beng
Profuse Bleeding in Young Women

(Some) young women invariably suffer from profuse uterine bleeding during the third month of pregnancy and subsequently have a miscarriage. People suppose (this to be due to) injuries by wrenching or contusion. Who would suspect that it is caused by indiscreet sexual intercourse? Naturally, the only appropriate treatment method is to mainly supplement the qi with the use of a small amount of blood-supplementing ingredients. The formula to use is ***Gu Qi Tang*** (Consolidate the Qi Decoction):

Radix Panacis Ginseng (*Ren Shen*), 1 *liang*
Rhizoma Atractylodis Macrocephalae (*Bai Zhu*), 5 *qian*, stir-fried with earth
Radix Coquitus Rehmanniae (*Shu Di*), 5 *qian*, steamed 9 times
Radix Angelicae Sinensis (*Dang Gui*), 3 *qian*, washed with wine
Sclerotium Poriae Cocoris (*Bai Fu Ling*), 2 *qian*
Radix Glycyrrhizae (*Gan Cao*), 1 *qian*
Cortex Eucommiae Ulmoidis (*Du Zhong*), 3 *qian*, char-fried
Fructus Corni Officinalis (*Shan Yu Rou*), 2 *qian*, steamed
Radix Polygalae Tenuifoliae (*Yuan Zhi*), 1 *qian*, cored
Fructus Schizandrae Chinensis (*Wu Wei Zi*), 10 pieces, stir-fried

Decoct in water and take. (After) 1 *ji*, bleeding is stopped; 10 *ji* taken in succession and a complete cure is effected. This formula consolidates the qi and simultaneously supplements the blood. (Thus,) it is able to make up the lost blood quickly and to hold back the blood on the verge of desertion. It not only treats abortive uterine bleeding but is specifically effective against all types of qi vacuity *beng lou*. Its subtlety of subtleties lies in its not (taking the trouble to) stop bleeding but (using) qi-supplementing ingredients to act as blood stoppers.[2]

[One should refrain from sexual intercourse during pregnancy. If one does not refrain from it, one will most probably abort even though one luckily escapes uterine bleeding. If one does not abort, the child to which one gives birth is difficult to rear. Take care! Practice abstention![3]]

Jiao Gan Xue Chu
(Sexual) Union Causing Bleeding

(Some) women engage in sexual intercourse which leads to flowing blood which does not stop. Though (this bleeding is) not so serious as profuse (uterine) bleeding or *xue beng*, if it continues throughout the year, typically both blood and qi will be injured. If it lasts for a long time, this will likely lead to worry due to withered blood and *jing bi* or menstrual block, (*i.e.*, amenorrhea). Such disease is brought on by *jing* essence

---

2 In Chinese medicine, if one states stopping bleeding or *zhi xue* as one of the treatment principles in a case, then one is expected to select and add at least some ingredients from the *zhi xue* or stop bleeding category of medicinals. However, this formula does not include any specifically *zhi xue* ingredients and yet, its net effect is to stop bleeding.

3 This opinion is based on the traditional Chinese concept of fetal education. According to this idea, the fetus is aware of its mother's experiences and is directly affected by them. These experiences shape the fetus' personality *in utero*. Therefore, a fetus exposed to sexual desire will grow up with strong desires of their own with the implication that that will make them hard to handle.

surging into the blood vessels during sexual intercourse during the very course of menstruation. *Jing* essence surging into the blood vessel causes temporary injury only, which ought to heal after the essence is discharged. Then why does the red run continually? It should be understood that the blood vessels are the tenderest of all and should be kept from injury by *jing* essence no matter what. To be on the safe side, conception in women must be implanted at a time when the blood vessels are clear. If *jing* essence is ejaculated into (the uterus/*bao gong*) when the menstrual flow is at high tide and about to gush out, the blood on the verge of leaving will turn back and withdraw. Thus, not only is there no possibility of fertilization to develop a fetus, but the *jing* is bound to gather and transform the blood. In the process of sexual intercourse, as the *yin* or sexual qi[4] touches the old, retained *jing*, due to the action of mutual sympathy, the old *jing* is inclined to come out and with it also exits the blood. The treatment method must be to free the qi of the *bao tai* in order to lead the old, gathered *jing* out. In addition, (one must also) introduce qi and essence supplementing medicinals. Thus injury of the blood vessels can be well mended. The formula to use is ***Yin Jing Zhi Xue Tang*** (Lead the Essence, Stop Bleeding Decoction):

Radix Panacis Ginseng (*Ren Shen*), 5 *qian*
Rhizoma Atractylodis Macrocephalae (*Bai Zhu*), 1 *qian*, stir-fried with earth
Sclerotium Poriae Cocoris (*Fu Ling*), 3 *qian*, skinned
Radix Coquitus Rehmanniae (*Shu Di*), 1 *liang*, steamed 9 times
Fructus Corni Officinalis (*Shan Yu Rou*), 5 *qian*, steamed
Rhizoma Carbonisata Zingiberis (*Hei Jiang*), 1 *qian*
Cortex Phellodendri (*Huang Bai*), 5 *fen*

---

4 The word here is *yin*. This *yin* not only means sex but also implies loose or licentious.

Herba Seu Flos Schizonepetae Tenuifoliae (*Jie Sui*), 3 *qian*
Semen Plantaginis (*Che Qian Zi*), 3 *qian*, stir-fried with wine

Decoct in water. Four *ji* taken in succession and a cure is effected; 10 *ji* prevent relapse. This formula employs Radix Panacis Ginseng and Rhizoma Atractylodis Macrocephalae to supplement the qi and Radix Coquitus Rehmanniae and Fructus Corni Officinalis to supplement the essence. Once essence and qi are made effulgent, the blood vessels become free flowing. Sclerotium Poriae Cocoris and Semen Plantaginis are introduced to disinhibit water and the portals. As water is disinhibited, the blood vessels are disinhibited too. Furthermore, Cortex Phellodendri is introduced as a conductor to lead (the other medicinals) directly into the blood vessels so as to lead the old *jing* out of them, while Herba Seu Flos Schizonepetae Tenuifoliae conducts the vanquished blood out of the blood vessels and charred Rhizoma Zingiberis stops up the openings of the blood vessels. As this one single formula has all the sophisticated efficacy of regulation and stoppage, it is capable of dispelling enduring disease and eliminating chronic afflictions. Nevertheless, it is necessary to refrain from sexual intercourse for three months lest what is damaged should incur a new wound or what is mended should incur a new injury. Otherwise the effect will work for the time being only. Be cautious about this! Try to be free from sexual desire!

Yu Jie Xue Beng
Depression Knotting Profuse Bleeding

(Some) women who are desperately depressed suffer from profuse (uterine) bleeding with dry mouth and tongue, thirst, retching, vomiting, and acid regurgitation. People all treat (such cases) as fire disease, sometimes successfully and sometimes not. Why is this? It is because they are ignorant of (the cause of) depression and knotting of the liver qi. The liver governs the storing of blood. Blood, therefore, binds or knots when the liver qi binds. Then how is it that uterine bleeding develops? The liver is impetuous by nature. When its qi becomes bound, it becomes more impetuous than ever, and when it very impetuous, blood cannot be stored. As a result, bleeding becomes unavoidable. The appropriate treatment method is to primarily open depression. However, only opening depression with no care to calming the liver makes the liver qi wide open. In consequence, liver fire burns even more intensely. What's more, this bleeding cannot then be stopped. The formula to use is ***Ping Gan Ka Yu Zhi Xue Tang*** (Level the Liver, Open Depression, Stop Bleeding Decoction):

Radix Albus Paeoniae Lactiflorae (*Bai Shao*), 1 *liang*, stir-fried with vinegar
Rhizoma Atractylodis Macrocephalae (*Bai Zhu*), 1 *liang*, stir-fried with earth
Radix Angelicae Sinensis (*Dang Gui*), 1 *liang*, washed with wine
Cortex Radicis Moutan (*Dan Pi*), 3 *qian*
Radix Pseudoginseng (*San Qi Geng*), 3 *qian*, powdered,
Radix Rehmanniae (*Sheng Di*), 3 *qian*, stir-fried with wine
Radix Glycyrrhizae (*Gan Cao*), 2 *qian*
Herba Seu Flos Carbonisatus Schizonepetae Tenuifoliae (*Hei Jie Sui*), 2 *qian*
Radix Bupleuri (*Chai Hu*), 1 *qian*

Decoct in water and take. One *ji* checks retching and vomiting; a second *ji* quenches dryness and thirst; (and) a fourth *ji* cures uterine bleeding. The subtlety of this formula lies in its ridding of all worry of blood accumulation and settling by using Radix Albus Paeoniae Lactiflorae to level the liver, Radix Bupleuri to open depression, and Rhizoma Atractylodis Macrocephalae to disinhibit the lumbus and navel. Because Herba Seu Flos Schizonepetae Tenuifoliae frees the flow of the channels and the connecting vessels, blood can enjoy a happy return. In addition, Cortex Radicis Moutan clears heat from the bone marrow and Radix Rehmanniae is further capable of clearing flames from the viscera and bowels. Radix Angelicae Sinensis and Radix Pseudoginseng stop bleeding together with supplementing the blood. Thus, it is only natural that depression and knotting are dispersed and that *xue beng* is stopped.

[It is even better to add 3 *qian* of charred Rhizoma Guanzhong (*Guan Zhong*) to this formula.]

Shan Die Xue Beng
Profuse Bleeding Due to Wrenching & Falling

(Some) women experience falls from a height or injuries from wrenching and contusion and hence discharge malign blood from below similar to *xue beng*. If, however, this is treated as uterine bleeding, harm rather than good is done. The signs of this pattern include tender spots which invariably give pain in response to pressure and, in long-standing cases, a withered, yellow facial complexion and a desiccated, emaciated appearance. (All this) is due to blood stasis, something incomparable to profuse uterine bleeding or *xue beng*. If (the physician) is not conscious of resolving stasis but instead employs supplementing and astringing, then blood stasis will attack inwards and pain will never cease. In consequence, new blood cannot be generated and old blood cannot be transformed. Is it not deplorable if (such a physician) does not come to realize (this mistake) to the end of his life? The treatment methods must be to move the blood to eliminate stasis and to quicken the blood to relieve pain. Thus bleeding will stop of itself and naturally be cured. The formula to use is ***Zhu Yu Zhi Xue Tang*** (Expel Stasis, Stop Bleeding Decoction):

Radix Rehmanniae (*Sheng Di*), 1 *liang*, stir-fried with wine

Radix Et Rhizoma Rhei (*Da Huang*), 3 *qian*
Radix Rubrus Paeoniae Lactiflorae (*Chi Shao*), 3 *qian*
Cortex Radicis Moutan (*Dan Pi*), 1 *qian*
Apex Radicis Angelicae Sinensis (*Dang Gui Wei*), 5 *qian*
Fructus Citri Seu Ponciri (*Zhi Qiao*), 5 *qian*, stir-fried
Plastrum Testudinis (*Gui Ban*), 3 *qian*, stir-fried with vinegar
Semen Pruni Persicae (*Tao Ren*), 10 pieces, soaked, fried, & mashed

Decoct in water and take. One *ji* will mitigate pain; a second *ji* will relieve it; a third *ji* will stop bleeding completely. No more doses are necessary. The subtlety of this formula lies in its ability to expel stasis in a sweeping way and stop bleeding miraculously by introducing, among blood-quickening (medicinals), stasis-precipitating agents as assistants. (Bleeding) due to falls, wrenching, or contusion is an external injury which transforms into an internal injury. Although it is not as serious as internal injury, the interior cannot be said to be only slightly injured since it has developed profuse bleeding. Then it may be questioned why stasis alone is treated without regard to the qi. It should be understood that falls, wrenching, or contusion are incomparable to external injury transformed from internal injury. While the root is still solid and impregnable, it is proper if only the branch disease is eliminated. Because of this, it is said that the branch should be treated in an acute case.

[This is also an appropriate treatment method for any type of spitting or retching of blood due to impact injury. To treat blood gathering in the stomach, it is proper to add 1 1/2 *qian* of Cortex Magnoliae Officinalis (*Chuan Hou Po*) stir-fried with ginger juice.]

Xue Hai Da Re Xue Beng Profuse Bleeding (Due to) Great Heat (in the) Sea of Blood

(Some) women never follow the path of (most) humans (*i.e.*, go in for sexual intercourse), but when their menstruation comes, it is like *xue beng* or profuse uterine bleeding. People suppose (this is due to) an injured uterus whose blood gets stirred by touching[5]. Who would suspect lack of consolidation of the uterus and the sea of blood due to greatly excessive heat? The womb or *zi gong* is situated under the *bao tai*[6] above which lies the *xue hai* or sea of blood. What is called the sea of blood is the penetrating vessel or *chong mai*. If the *chong mai* is too cold, blood is depleted. If it is too hot, blood boils (over). The cause of *xue beng* is none other than excessively great heat in the *chong mai*. However, since it is due to the heat of the penetrating vessel, (such) uterine bleeding should be perpetual rather than intermittent. Then why does it not arise till after sexual intercourse? Does it really have nothing to do with liver/wood? The spleen, when strong, is able to contain the blood. The liver, when calm or level, is able to store the blood. Before sexual intercourse, imperial and ministerial fires are quiet and tranquil. Therefore, if only the *chong mai* is hot, blood will not run out. When the sexual urge is felt, the womb is wide open and imperial and ministerial fires begin to stir. Heat invites heat, while similar qi appeal to each other. (Thus,) they both

---

5 This implies that though the woman does not usually indulge in sex, this *xue beng* occurs after a sexual encounter.

6 Usually, one thinks of the *zi gong* or fetal palace as being one and the same as the *bao tai* or uterus/fetus. Here it apparently refers to something other than that. It may mean a nonsubstantial, functional entity where the *ren, chong,* and *du* vessels originate and which governs reproduction in females.

begin to stir all of a sudden and agitate the essence chamber. Hence the sea of blood overflows with such an uncheckable momentum that the liver is no longer able to store (the blood), while the spleen is unable to contain it. As a result, the menstrual flow follows sexual intercourse immediately as an echo responds to sound. Nothing but fire is capable of producing such a disease. The treatment methods must be to enrich yin and downbear fire so as to clear the sea of blood and to harmonize the womb. Thus, an otherwise life long disease can be stopped in its tracks. This, however, can only be realized after three months of refraining from sexual intercourse. The formula to use is ***Qing Hai Wan*** (Clear the Sea Pills):

Radix Coquitus Rehmanniae (*Da Shu Di*), 1 *jin*, steamed 9 times
Fructus Corni Officinalis (*Shan Yu Rou*), 10 *liang*, steamed
Radix Dioscoreae Oppositae (*Shan Yao*), 10 *liang*, stir-fried
Cortex Radicis Moutan (*Dan Pi*), 10 *liang*
Fructus Schizandrae Chinensis (*Bei Wu Wei*), 2 *liang*, stir-fried
Tuber Ophiopogonis Japonicae (*Mai Dong Rou*), 10 *liang*, skinned
Rhizoma Atractylodis Macrocephalae (*Bai Zhu*), 1 *jin*, stir-fried with earth
Radix Albus Paeoniae Lactiflorae (*Bai Shao*), 1 *jin*, stir-fried with wine
Os Draconis (*Long Gu*), 2 *liang*
Cortex Radicis Lycii (*Di Gu Pi*), 10 *liang*
Folium Mori Albi (*Gan Sang Ye*), 1 *jin*
Radix Scrophulariae Ningpoensis (*Yuan Shen*), 1 *jin*
Radix Glehniae Littoralis (*Sha Shen*), 10 *liang*
Herba Dendrobii (*Shi Hu*), 10 *liang*

Fourteen ingredients altogether (are) all to be powdered, mixed together, and prepared with heated honey in (the form of) pills the size of phoenix tree seeds. Take with boiled water in the morning and evening, 5 *qian* each time. The cure will be effected after half a year. This formula supplements yin without (having to) worry about causing insecurity and provocation. It also concentrates the blood without (causing) affliction by cold or cooling. Each single day seems of no significance (while taking this medicine) but, when counted by the month, (the result) is more than sufficient. Little by little without notice, the womb is cooled and the sea of blood consequently becomes consolidated. Suppose the end were emphasized while the root was given no importance and medicinals, such as Crinis Carbonisatus (*Fa Hui*), Alum (*Bai Fan*), Rhizoma Carbonisata Coptidis Chinensis (*Huang Lian Tan*), and Galla Rhi Chinensis (*Wi Bei Zi*), were introduced for external treatment of the private parts. In that case, it is likely that the more astringing were applied, the more blood would pour out and that this would certainly lead to death in the end. How can caution not be taken?

Chapter 3

Tiao Jing Balancing the Menses

Jing Shui Xian Qi Menstruation Ahead of Schedule

(Some) women have menstruation ahead of schedule (*i.e.*, early menstruation) with excessive flow. People suppose this is (due to) extremely hot blood. Who would suspect too effulgent water and fire in the kidneys? When fire is too effulgent, blood gets hot. When water is too effulgent, the blood becomes abundant. (Therefore,) this is a disease of abundance rather than insufficiency. It seems that no medication is needed and a happy event is to be.[1] However, once abundance goes beyond limit, the womb becomes too hot, making it difficult to conceive regardless (of this abundance). What's worse, there is a danger of scorching and drying up the *jing* of males. Then is it not a *ji ji* way[2] to apply reduction to what is superabundant? It is true that superabundant fire cannot be left unattended, but in no circumstances should water be made insufficient. Therefore, the treatment method is just to clear

---

1 This is a euphemism for pregnancy.

2 This again refers to the same hexagram mentioned in note 11 on page 11 above.

fire a little without draining water. The formula to use is ***Qing Jing San*** (Clear Menstruation Powder):

Cortex Radicis Moutan (*Dan Pi*), 3 *qian*
Cortex Radicis Lycii (*Di Gu Pi*), 5 *qian*
Radix Albus Paeoniae Lactiflorae (*Bai Shao*), 3 *qian*, stir-fried with wine
Radix Coquitus Rehmanniae (*Da Shu Di*), 3 *qian*, steamed 9 times
Herba Artemisiae Apiaceae (*Qing Hao*), 2 *qian*
Sclerotium Poriae Cocoris (*Bai Fu Ling*), 1 *qian*
Cortex Phellodendri (*Huang Bai*), 5 *fen*, soaked in salt water, then stir-fried

Decoct in water and take. Two *ji* will certainly put down the fire. Though it is composed of medicinals which clear fire, this is a formula to enrich water. Fire is drained but water is not. The formula reduces (in one way) while boosting (in another).

There is also early menstruation with only a dot of bleeding. People suppose this to be (due to) extreme hot blood. Who would suspect effulgent fire in the kidneys with depletion of yin water? And, why should there be one classification of vacuity and another of repletion when only one and the same (disease, *i.e.)*, advanced menstruation, is concerned? It is most difficult to balance the menstruation in women. If one does not discriminate finely and minutely, the use of medicinals seldom have (their intended) effect. (The period being) early (indicates) raging fire qi. While the excessive amount is (a manifestation of) water qi. Therefore, early menstruation excessive in amount means fire/heat with superabundant water. While early menstruation scant in amount means fire heat with insufficient water. If (one) attributes all advanced menstruation whatsoever to excessive fire and knows nothing but to drain fire without supplementing water or to drain both water and fire, can one not make the disease worse? (In this case,) the treatment method is to exclusively supplement water without draining fire. Once water becomes abundant, fire is automatically extinguished. This is also one of the *ji ji* ways. The formula to use is ***Liang Di Tang*** (Two *Di* Decoction):

Radix Rehmanniae (*Da Sheng Di*), 1 *liang*, stir-fried with wine
Radix Scrophulariae Ningpoensis (*Yuan Shen*), 1 *liang*
Radix Albus Paeoniae Lactiflorae (*Bai Shao Yao*), 5 *qian*, stir-fried
Tuber Ophiopogonis Japonicae (*Mai Dong Rou*), 5 *qian*, skinned
Cortex Radicis Lycii (*Di Gu Pi*), 3 *qian*
Gelatinum Corii Asini (*E Jiao*), 3 *qian*

Decoct in water and take. Four *ji* (and) the menstruation is balanced. The purpose of including Cortex Radicis Lycii and Radix Rehmanniae is to clear heat inside the bones which is the result of heat in the kidney channel. When the bone marrow is cleared, kidney qi naturally is cleared and (this) without damaging the stomach qi. This is a clever treatment. Furthermore, all the ingredients introduced are purely medicinals which supplement water. Once water becomes effulgent, fire is naturally extinguished and rectified. Cross-referencing this and the last formula will surely prevent contrary treatment of early menstruations (of any type).

Jing Shui Hou Qi
Menstruation Behind Schedule

(Some) women have menstruation behind schedule (or delayed menstrual flow) in great amounts. People suppose (such cases are) a blood vacuity disease. Who suspects anything other than blood vacuity? As far as late periods are concerned, (however,) there is a difference (depending upon) the amount of flow. Therefore, one should not adhere to a one-sided view (treating all late periods without further classification). Late periods with a small amount of flow indicate cold, insufficient blood. While late periods with a great quantity of flow demonstrate cold, superabundant blood. The menstrual flow originates in the kidneys and the blood which has run all through the five viscera and six bowels returns (to them). Because of this, when the menstrual flow appears, the blood in the various channels all flows toward and joins (the menstrual flow). (Thus,) because of the menstrual flow, the gates (of the body) open but may fail to close quick enough. Consequently, the blood of the various channels may take advantage of these gates still being ajar in order to come out. Once (part of the) blood has run out, the blood becomes insufficient. The appropriate treatment method is to incorporate warming and dissipation into supplementation. It is wrong to declare that delayed menstruation is invariably ascribed to insufficiency. The formula to use is ***Wen Jing She Xue Tang*** (Warm the Menses/Channels, Contain the Blood Decoction):

Radix Coquitus Rehmanniae (*Da Shu Di*), 1 *liang*, steamed 9 times
Radix Albus Paeoniae Lactiflorae (*Bai Shao*), 1 *liang*, stir-fried with wine
Rhizoma Ligustici Wallichii (*Chuan Xiong*), 5 *qian*, washed with wine
Rhizoma Atractylodis Macrocephalae (*Bai Zhu*), 5 *qian*, stir-fried with earth
Radix Bupleuri (*Chai Hu*), 5 *fen*
Fructus Schizandrae Chinensis (*Wu Wei Zi*), 3 *fen*
Radix Dipsaci (*Xu Duan*), 1 *qian*
Cortex Cinnamomi (*Rou Gui*), 5 *fen*, sorted & ground

Decoct in water and take. Three *ji* (and) the menstruation is balanced. This formula greatly supplements the essence and blood of the liver, kidneys, and spleen with Cortex Cinnamomi included to dispel cold and Radix Bupleuri to resolve depression. Thus, in the midst of supplementing, it dissipates or scatters. But, though it scatters, it does not consume qi. In the midst of supplementing, it (also) drains. But, though it drains, it does not reduce yin. Therefore, its supplementation brings nothing but profit and its warming is its own effect. Because of this, these are wonderful medicinals for balancing menstruation and an immortal's elixir for containing the blood. It is applicable to all types of late or delayed periods. In case of insufficient *yuan* or original qi, 1 or 2 *qian* of Radix Panacis Ginseng (*Ren Shen*) can be added.

Jing Shui Xian Hou Wu Ding Qi
Menstruation Early, Late, At No Fixed Intervals

(Some) women have menstruation which is interrupted or appears at irregular intervals. People suppose (such cases) as one of qi and blood vacuity. Who would suspect depression and knotting of liver qi? The menstrual flow has its source in the kidneys. Because the liver is the child of the kidneys, when the liver is depressed, the kidneys are also depressed. When the kidneys are depressed, their qi is surely not perfusive. The advance, delay, or interruption in continuity (of menstruation) are the very indicators of free (*tong*) or blocked (*bi*) kidneys. It may be argued that such a condition can not arise should the kidneys not respond if liver qi becomes depressed. It should be understood, (however,) that mother and child are concerned with each other. When the child is ill, the mother must worry and have sympathy. When the liver is depressed, the kidneys cannot help cherishing compassion. Opening or blocking of the liver qi means departure or preservation of the kidney qi. There should be no doubt that such a causal relationship exists. The appropriate treatment method is to soothe the depression of the liver which is followed by opening the depression of kidney qi. Once the depression of the liver and kidneys is opened, menstruation will naturally become regular. The formula to use is ***Ding Jing Tang*** (Fix the Menses Decoction):

Semen Cuscutae (*Tu Si Zi*), 1 *liang*, stir-fried with wine
Radix Albus Paeoniae Lactiflorae (*Bai Shao*), 1 *liang*, stir-fried with wine
Radix Angelicae Sinensis (*Dang Gui*), 1 *liang*, washed with wine
Radix Coquitus Rehmanniae (*Da Shu Di*), 5 *qian*, steamed 9 times
Radix Dioscoreae Oppositae (*Shan Yao*), 5 *qian*, stir-fried
Sclerotium Poriae Cocoris (*Bai Fu Ling*), 3 *qian*
Herba Seu Flos Schizonepetae Tenuifoliae (*Jie Sui*), 2 *qian*, char-fried
Radix Bupleuri (*Chai Hu*), 5 *fen*

Decoct in water and take. Two *ji* (and) the menses is cleared; 4 *ji* (and) menstruation becomes regular. This is a formula composed of medicinals to soothe the liver and kidney qi instead of freeing the menstrual flow. Its ingredients supplement the essence of liver and kidneys instead of disinhibiting water. Once, however, the liver and kidney qi is soothed, their essence is freed, and, when liver and kidney essence is effulgent, water is (automatically) disinhibited. The subtlety lies in its effectiveness being obtained without employing what is (otherwise believed to be) effective.

[The above three sections on balancing menstruation are discriminating, clear discussions and (give) subtle, sophisticated formulas. However, in some particular cases with (complications of) external invasion (*wai gan*) or internal injury (*nei shang*), these formulas may not prove so effective. Add 1 *qian* of Folium Perillae Frutescentis (*Su Ye*) in case of external invasion, 2 *qian* of stir-fried Massa Medica Fermentata (*Shen Qu*) in case of internal injury, and 2 *qian* of stir-fried Fructus Crataegi (*Shan Zha Rou*) in addition to Massa Medica Fermentata in case of meat-type food accumulation and stagnation. Variations should be made in accordance with the clinical manifestations. In case of liver qi depression, *Xiao Yao San* (Rambling Powder) should be prescribed as the basis. In case of heat, add charred Fructus Gardeniae Jasminoidis (*Zhi Zi*) and Cortex Radicis Moutan (*Dan Pi*) to form *Jia Wei Xiao Yao San* (Rambling Powder with Added Flavors).]

Jing Shui Shu Yue Yi Xing
Menstruation Comes Once Every Several Months

(Some) women have menstruation appearing quite regularly (only) once every several months, neither earlier nor later, and with constant amounts of flow that never vary. People all consider (such cases) aberrant, but, practically (speaking), there is nothing abnormal about it. (This may be seen) in healthy persons without any depletion or damage of qi and blood. However, (the fact) that it is also often seen in persons with detriment to life done by over-indulgence in sexual affairs makes it necessary to design a formula to rescue them. This formula is called ***Zhu Xian Dan*** (Assisting Immortal Elixir):

Sclerotium Poriae Cocoris (*Bai Fu Ling*), 5 *qian*
Pericarpium Citri Reticulatae (*Chen Pi*), 5 *qian*
Rhizoma Atractylodis Macrocephalae (*Bai Zhu*), 3 *qian*, stir-fried with earth
Radix Albus Paeoniae Lactiflorae (*Bai Shao*), 3 *qian*, stir-fried with wine
Radix Dioscoreae Oppositae (*Shan Yao*), 3 *qian*, stir-fried

Semen Cuscutae (*Tu Si Zi*), 2 *qian*, stir-fried with wine
Cortex Eucommiae Ulmoidis (*Du Zhong*), 1 *qian*, char-fried
Radix Glycyrrhizae (*Gan Cao*), 1 *qian*

Decoct in river water and take. If the condition remains the same as before after having taken 4 *ji*, no more should be administered. This formula has indeed a subtle mechanism in tempered supplementation. It fortifies the spleen and boosts the kidneys without bringing about stagnation, and it resolves depression and clears phlegm without resulting in drainage. Not damaging natural qi and blood is the great method in balancing menstruation. What is the point of employing other medicinals in the hope of freeing the menstrual flow?

Lao Nian Jing Shui Fu Xing
Recurrent Menstruation in Old Women

(Some) old women more than 50 or even 60 or 70 years of age suddenly resume menstruation with purple blood clots or dribbling red blood. People may comment that recurrent menstruation in old women is a sign of rejuvenation. Who would suspect that this is profuse (uterine) bleeding or *xue beng* in progress? When women are above 7 times 7 years old, their *tian gui*[3] is exhausted. Without having taken medicinals to succor yin or supplement yang, how can their essence be full enough to transform into menses the way a young woman's does? In any case, menstruation appearing at a time when it should not is the result of the liver failing to store (blood) and the spleen failing to govern (it). It is caused either by essence unduly drained so as to stir the *ming men zhi huo* or fire of the gate of life or by such severe depression of qi as to

3 *Tian gui* literally means heavenly water. It generally refers to the human reproductive function in females.

burst into a dragon-thunderous flame. Two fires[4] break out simultaneously so that blood runs in a rampant way. It seems to be but is not menstruation. To stop bleeding immediately in such a pattern, there is no other choice but to greatly supplement the qi and blood of the liver and the spleen. The formula to use is ***An Lao Tang*** (Calm the Aged Decoction):

Radix Panacis Ginseng (*Ren Shen*), 1 *liang*
Radix Astragali Seu Hedysari (*Huang Qi*), 1 *liang*, use raw
Radix Coquitus Rehmanniae (*Da Shu Di*), 1 *liang*, steamed 9 times
Rhizoma Atractylodis Macrocephalae (*Bai Zhu*), 5 *qian*, stir-fried with earth
Radix Angelicae Sinensis (*Dang Gui*), 5 *qian*, washed with wine
Fructus Corni Officinalis (*Shan Yu*), 5 *qian*, steamed
Gelatinum Corii Asini (*E Jiao*), 1 *qian*, stir-fried with powdered clam shell
Herba Seu Flos Carbonisatus Schizonepetae Tenuifoliae (*Hei Jie Sui*), 1 *qian*
Radix Glycyrrhizae (*Gan Cao*), 1 *qian*
Rhizoma Cyperi Rotundi (*Xiang Fu*), 5 *fen*, stir-fried with wine
Exidia Auricula Judae (*Mu Er Tan*), 1 *qian*, (charred)

Decoct in water and take. One *ji* will effect reduction; a second *ji* will effect (a more) marked reduction; a fourth *ji* will reduce (the bleeding) to naught; a tenth *ji* will effect a complete cure. This formula supplements and boosts the qi of the liver and the spleen. Once qi is abundant, blood is naturally generated and contained. What is particularly subtle about this formula is its great supplementation of kidney water. Once water is abundant, liver qi is naturally soothed, and once the liver qi is

---

4 Two fires refer to vacuity fire from lack of kidney yin and liver fire due to stagnant qi transforming into depressive heat. These two fires are then *xiang sheng* or mutually engendering.

soothed, the spleen naturally is nurtured. Since the liver is that which stores (the blood) and the spleen is that which governs it, how can leakage occur and where is the cause for worry about profuse (uterine) bleeding?

[Add 1 *qian* of Rhizoma Guanzhong (*Guan Zhong*); char powder, add to the other medicinals, and take for an even better effect.]

Jing Shui Hu Lai Hu Duan Shi Teng Shi Zhi Menstruation Suddenly Comes, Suddenly Ceases, Sometimes Pain, Sometimes Stops[5]

(Some) women have menstruation which suddenly comes and suddenly ceases. Sometimes there is pain and sometimes it stops. There may (also) be alternating fever and chills. People suppose (this is due to) congelation of blood. Who would suspect unsoothed liver qi? The liver which stores blood belongs to wood. It hates wind and cold most of all. In the course of menstruation, women's *cou li* or interstices are wide open. If they happen to be caught in wind or attacked by cold, liver qi will be blocked and subsequently the passageways of the menstrual flow are all blocked as well. As a result, the interstices and channels and connecting vessels all become nondiffusive and thus fever and chills arise. When the qi travels in the yang phase, heat is generated. When it travels in the yin phase, cold is generated. This, however, is but a slight case of (external) invasion. The more serious the external invasion of wind cold is, the deeper the responding internal hot qi penetrates. There are even patterns where this hot qi

---

5 *I.e.*, the pain stops.

penetrates the blood chamber to cause mania-like disease. If merely alternating fever and chills are present, wind cold is not too serious and heat has not penetrated deep. The appropriate treatment methods are to supplement the blood in the liver, relieve depression, and dissipate or scatter wind. In this way, the disease will be cured in no time. This is an example illustrating the saying that blood should be treated to treat wind and that wind dies down of itself once blood is harmonized. The formula to use is ***Jia Wei Si Wu Tang*** (Added Flavors Four Ingredient Decoction):

Radix Coquitus Rehmanniae (*Da Shu Di*), 1 *liang*, steamed 9 times
Radix Albus Paeoniae Lactiflorae (*Bai Shao*), 5 *qian*, stir-fried with wine
Radix Angelicae Sinensis (*Dang Gui*), 5 *qian*, washed with wine
Rhizoma Ligustici Wallichii (*Chuan Xiong*), 3 *qian*, washed with wine
Rhizoma Atractylodis Macrocephalae (*Bai Zhu*), 5 *qian*, stir-fried with earth
Cortex Radicis Moutan (*Fen Dan Pi*), 3 *qian*
Rhizoma Corydalis Yanhusuo (*Yuan Hu*), 1 *qian*, stir-fried with wine
Radix Glycyrrhizae (*Gan Cao*), 1 *qian*
Radix Bupleuri (*Chai Hu*), 1 *qian*

Decoct in water and take. This formula employs *Si Wu* to enrich the yin blood of the spleen and stomach, Radix Bupleuri, Radix Albus Paeoniae Lactiflorae, and Cortex Radicis Moutan to diffuse the wind depression of the liver channel, and Radix Glycyrrhizae, Rhizoma Atractylodis Macrocephalae, and Rhizoma Corydalis Yanhusuo to disinhibit the lumbus and navel to relieve abdominal pain. (The strength of these medicinals) works in both the exterior and the interior and finds its way into both the channels and the connecting vessels. If the formula is used in an appropriate way, its effect will appear as (quickly as an echo follows a) sound.

[Add Herba Seu Flos Schizonepetae Tenuifoliae (*Jing Jie Sui*), slightly charred, 1 *qian* for a better effect.]

Jing Shui Wei Lai Fu Xian Teng Menstruation Not Yet Arrived Preceded by Abdominal Ache

(Some) women have several days of abdominal pain prior to menstruation which (then comes) usually with amounts of dark purple blood clots. People suppose (this is due to) extreme cold. Who would suspect fire failing to transform due to extreme heat? The liver, which belongs to wood, contains fire within it. So long as it is soothed, it is free and uninhibited. But when it is depressed, it becomes inert. Therefore, when the menstrual flow is about to start, the liver fails to respond and consequently its qi is oppressed and hindered, (thus) producing pain. Nonetheless, the jammed up menses cannot be stored in the interior while depressive fire in the liver is burning and forcing it from within to come out. With the discharge of the menses, the fire drains out in a tempestuous way. The dark purple color is a sign of the battle between water and fire, and the forming of clots reveals the work of simmering fire. That the menses is not as the menses should be is (due to) righteous and evil fire struggling in the interior. The appropriate treatment method is to greatly drain fire from the liver. But solely draining it without resolving liver depression only removes the branch of the heat but not its root. What good is that? The formula to use is ***Xuan Yu Tong Jing*** *Tang* (Diffuse Depression, Free the Menses Decoction):

Radix Albus Paeoniae Lactiflorae (*Bai Shao*), 5 *qian*, stir-fried with wine
Radix Angelicae Sinensis (*Dang Gui*), 5 *qian*, washed with wine
Cortex Radicis Moutan (*Dan Pi*), 5 *qian*
Fructus Gardeniae Jasminoidis (*Shan Zhi Zi*), 3 *qian*, stir-fried
Semen Sinapis Albae (*Bai Jie Zi*), 2 *qian*, stir-fried & ground
Radix Bupleuri (*Chai Hu*), 1 *qian*
Rhizoma Cyperi Rotundi (*Xiang Fu*), 1 *qian*, stir-fried with wine
Tuber Curcumae (*Chuan Yu Jin*), 1 *qian*, stir-fried with vinegar
Radix Scutellariae Baicalensis (*Huang Qin*), 1 *qian*, stir-fried with wine
Radix Glycyrrhizae (*Sheng Gan Cao*), 1 *qian*

Decoct in water. After 4 *ji* taken in succession, the next menstruation will for sure not be preceded by abdominal pain. This formula supplements liver blood to resolve liver depression and disinhibits liver qi to downbear liver fire. Because of this, it works swiftly.

Xing Jing Hou Shao Fu Teng Tong Menstruation Followed by Lower Abdominal Aching & Pain

(Some) women have lower abdominal pain following menstruation. People suppose (this is due to) qi and blood vacuity. Who would suspect dried up kidney qi? The menstrual flow is the heavenly true water. It is always the case with the menses that when it is full, it spills and when it is vacuous, it is shut (blocked). Then why is vacuity capable of producing pain? The reason is that once it becomes vacuous, kidney water is unable to generate wood. Then liver/wood is bound to restrain spleen/earth. This struggle between wood and earth invariably gives rise to qi counterflow. Therefore, pain is produced. The treatment methods must be to soothe liver qi as the key and, in addition, to introduce certain medicinals to supplement the kidneys. When water is made abundant, liver qi is boosted and becomes calm. So long as liver qi is calm, counterflow qi is automatically normalized. Then what aching and pain can there be? The formula to use is ***Tiao Gan Tang*** (Balance the Liver Decoction):

Radix Dioscoreae Oppositae (*Shan Yao*), 5 *qian*, stir-fried
Gelatinum Corii Asini (*E Jiao*), 3 *qian*, stir-fried with wheat flour
Radix Angelicae Sinensis (*Dang Gui*), 3 *qian*, washed with wine
Radix Albus Paeoniae Lactiflorae (*Bai Shao*), 3 *qian*, stir-fried with wine
Fructus Corni Officinalis (*Shan Zhu Rou*), 3 *qian*, well-steamed
Radix Morindae Officinalis (*Ba Ji*), 1 *qian*, soaked in salt water
Radix Glycyrrhizae (*Gan Cao*), 1 *qian*

Decoct in water and take. This formula levels and balances the liver qi in a tempered way. It is not only able to reverse qi counterflow but is also good at relieving depressive pain. It is an ideal formula to balance and regulate postmenstrual disorders, not a specific formula merely to treat postmenstrual pain.

[These (two) formulas for abdominal pain prior to and after menstruation are quite miraculous, and they should not be modified. In case there are complications, these formulas should be used as the basis and (then) they can be expanded with certain medicinals. However, no one ingredient is allowed to be deleted from them.]

Jing Qian Fu Teng Tu Xue
Abdominal Aching & Vomiting of Blood Preceding Menstruation

(Some) women have sudden abdominal pain and vomit blood one or two days before menstruation. People suppose (this to be due to) extreme fire/heat. Who would suspect counterflow of liver qi? Because the liver is the most impetuous of all (the organs) by nature, its (flow) needs to be normal and should never be counterflow. When (its flow is) normal, its qi is calm. While, if it is counterflow, its qi becomes agitated and stirred up. Blood always follows suit, *(i.e.,* it always acts in response to qi). When qi is calm, blood is calm. When qi is stirred up, blood is stirred up. There is nothing odd about this correspondence. It may be questioned how the menses can follow the blood and move in such a reckless way that it eventually comes out from the mouth, since menstrual counterflow is ascribed to the kidneys rather than the liver. Is it because the liver fails to store blood? Or, is it because the kidneys refuse to receive the qi? It should be understood that the fire of the *shao yin,* impetuous as a galloping horse, can surge straight up once aided by liver fire. It moves so forcefully that it is quite easy for it to reverse the menses to bleed (from above). It is not necessary for the liver to fail in storing blood to cause the pattern of *tu xue* or vomiting blood. However, vomiting blood of this type differs from that of the various channels in that the latter is brought about by internal injury, while menstrual counterflow blood vomiting is caused by the provocation of internal spillage. (However,) in spite of this tremendous difference, all types of blood vomiting have in common qi counterflow underneath. (Therefore,) the appropriate treatment method would seem to be to level the liver to normalize the qi with no need to enrich essence to supplement the kidneys. (But,) blood vomiting due to menstrual counterflow, though not incurring loss of blood in large amounts, most probably causes very serious damage to the kidneys due to the repeated reversion (of the menses). On that account, the only appropriate method cannot but be to carry out qi-normalization through kidney supplementation. The formula to use is ***Shun Jing Tang*** (Normalize the Menses Decoction):

Radix Angelicae Sinensis (*Dang Gui*), 5 *qian*, washed with wine
Radix Coquitus Rehmanniae (*Da Shu Di*), 5 *qian*, steamed 9 times
Radix Albus Paeoniae Lactiflorae (*Bai Shao*), 2 *qian*, stir-fried with wine
Cortex Radicis Moutan (*Dan Pi*), 5 *qian*
Sclerotium Poriae Cocoris (*Bai Fu Ling*), 3 *qian*
Radix Glehniae Littoralis (*Sha Shen*), 3 *qian*
Herba Seu Flos Carbonisatus Schizonepetae Tenuifoliae (*Hei Jie Sui*), 3 *qian*

Decoct in water and take. One *ji* (and) vomiting of blood is checked; a second *ji* (and) the menses is normalized; 10 *ji* prevent relapse. Within this formula for supplementing the kidneys and balancing the menses are used ingredients to return blood back to the menses. This is a method for harmonizing the blood, but, practically (speaking,) it is also a method for normalizing the qi. If there is no liver counterflow, kidney qi will automatically become normal. (And,) when kidney qi is normal, what kind of menstrual counterflow can there be?

[Vomiting of blood is often seen in women in the prime of life. It should not be treated as a consumption pattern or *lao zheng*. Otherwise, the counterflow of liver qi is bound to get worse and, consequently, (what began) not as a consumption pattern will, in actuality, become one. It is even better if 1 *qian* of Radix Rubiae Cordifoliae (*Qian Cao*) and 8 *fen* of Radix Achyranthis Bidentatae (*Huai Niu Xi*) are added to this formula.]

Jing Shui Jiang Lai Qi Xia Xian Teng Tong Aching & Pain Below the Umbilicus Before the Period is About to Come

(Some) women have aching below their umbilicus 3-5 days just before their period is about to come. The pain may be lancinating or there may be alternating fever and chills with the menstrual flow similar to black soybean juice. People all suppose (this to be due to) extreme blood heat. Who would suspect that it is due to the struggle between cold and dampness in the lower burner? Cold and dampness are both (species of) evil qi. Women have their *chong* and *ren* vessels in the lower burner. The *chong mai* is the sea of blood, while the *ren mai,* which governs the *bao tai,* is the blood chamber or *xue shi.* These two vessels both like or desire the free flow of righteous qi but hate the invasion of evil qi. The menstrual flow comes out from these two vessels. But if cold and dampness fill them, internal disturbance ensues and the struggle between these two evils provokes pain. As these evils become more and more exuberant, the righteous qi becomes (more) debilitated day by day. Cold qi generates turbidity. The black discharge similar to black soybean juice is like a sign of cold water in the north. The treatment methods are to disinhibit dampness and warm cold to eliminate the disturbing evil qi from the *chong* and *ren.* Thus, the affliction of aching and pain below the umbilicus is relieved. The formula to use is ***Wen Qi Hua Shi Tang*** (Warm the Umbilicus, Transform Dampness Decoction):

Rhizoma Atractylodis Macrocephalae (*Bai Zhu*), 1 *liang,* stir-fried with earth
Sclerotium Poriae Cocoris (*Bai Fu Ling*), 3 *qian*
Radix Dioscoreae Oppositae (*Shan Yao*), 5 *qian,* stir-fried

Radix Morindae Officinalis (*Ba Ji Rou*), 5 *qian*, soaked in salt water
Semen Dolichoris Lablabis (*Bian Dou*), stir-fried, pounded, 3 *qian*
Semen Ginkgonis Bilobae (*Bai Guo*), 10 pieces, pounded
Semen Nelumbinis Nuciferae (*Jian Lian Zi*), 30 pieces with the core preserved

Decoct in water and take. (This formula) should, however, be administered 10 days prior to menstruation. Four *ji* will dispel the evil qi and succeed in balancing the menses, (thus) making conception possible as well. This formula is composed of Rhizoma Atractylodis Macrocephalae as the ruler to disinhibit the qi of the lumbus and navel, Radix Morindae Officinalis and Semen Ginkgonis Bilobae to free the flow of the conception vessel, and Semen Dolichoris Lablabis, Radix Dioscoreae Oppositae, and Semen Nelumbinis Nuciferae to protect the penetrating vessel. Thus, cold and dampness are wiped out and menstruation is automatically balanced so as to make conception possible. If this abdominal pain is mistaken for a hot disease and accordingly cool and cold medicinals are used without warrant, then the *chong* and *ren* will become vacuous and cold. The sea of blood would then become an icy sea and the blood chamber would become an icy chamber. Pregnancy would of course be hardly possible. And how long could even the pain be relieved?

[With regard to the qi of the penetrating and the conception vessels, it is proper to use flow-freeing but not downbearing (medicinals). Therefore, Rhizoma Atractylodis (*Cang Zhu*) and Semen Coicis Lachryma-jobi (*Yi Ren*) are not used to transform dampness. This (also) should be taken into consideration in similar cases.]

Jing Shui Guo Duo
Excessive Menstruation

(Some) women have a menstrual flow which is excessive in amount, one period following in the wake of another, with a withered, yellow facial complexion, generalized fatigue, and serious languor. People suppose (this to be due to) heat and superabundance of blood. Who would suspect blood too vacuous to return to the channels?[6] Only when blood is effulgent should the menses become abundant and when blood is vacuous, the menses should (seemingly) dwindle. However, here, on the contrary, menstrual flow is said to be abundant due to blood vacuity. How to explain this? It should be understood that if the blood, however effulgent, returns to the channels, the menses does not increase but, if the blood, however debilitated, fails to return to channels, the menses does not decrease. People nowadays attribute excessive menstrual flow to effulgent blood (indiscriminately) whenever it is met. This accounts for the oft-occurring failure in its treatment. Suppose excessive menstrual flow did mean effulgent blood. The constitution would certainly then be strong, the menstrual flow would come to a clear stop in due course, and subsequently the qi would be restored to normal. Then what makes one period follow in the wake of another, and what makes for the fatigue and languor? Only when the cause of excessive menstrual flow is blood vacuity, can menstruation occur time and again and do overwhelmingly extreme languor and weakness ensue. As blood is reduced, essence is dispersed, marrow becomes vacuous within the bones, and lustre is unable to appear on the face. The appro-

---

6 The word *jing* here is the same as used for both the channels and the menses. Therefore, this might also be translated as the blood being too vacuous to return to the menses. However, that would make little sense in this context.

priate treatment method is to greatly supplement blood and conduct it back to the channels. Thus, how can the problem of one period following in the wake of another persist any longer? The formula to use is *Jia Jian Si Wu Tang* (Modified Four Ingredient Decoction):

Radix Coquitus Rehmanniae (*Da Shu Di*), 1 *liang*, steamed 9 times
Radix Albus Paeoniae Lactiflorae (*Bai Shao*), 3 *qian*, stir-fried with wine
Radix Angelicae Sinensis (*Dang Gui*), 5 *qian*, washed with wine
Rhizoma Ligustici Wallichii (*Chuan Xiong*), 2 *qian*, washed with wine
Rhizoma Atractylodis Macrocephalae (*Bai Zhu*), 5 *qian*, stir-fried with earth
Herba Seu Flos Carbonisata Schizonepetae Tenuifoliae (*Hei Jie Sui*), 3 *qian*
Fructus Corni Officinalis (*Shan Yu*) 3 *qian*, steamed
Radix Dipsaci (*Xu Duan*), 1 *qian*
Radix Glycyrrhizae (*Gan Cao*), 1 *qian*

Decoct in water and take. Four *ji* (and) the blood is returned to the channels. After the tenth *ji*, add 3 *qian* of Radix Panacis Ginseng (*Ren Shen*) and administer 10 more *ji*. Then the next menstrual flow will stop in due time. *Si Wu Tang* is a divine composition for supplementing the blood. Rhizoma Atractylodis Macrocephalae and Herba Seu Flos Carbonisatus Schizonepetae Tenuifoliae are included to incorporate disinhibition into supplementation; Fructus Corni Officinalis and Radix Dipsaci to incorporate moving into stopping; and Radix Glycyrrhizae is included to balance and harmonize the other ingredients. Thus blood is made abundant and returns to the channels and, when it returns to the channels, it becomes automatically tranquil.

[Herba Seu Flos Carbonisatus Schizonepetae Tenuifoliae is able to lead blood back to the channels. This formula is perfectly miraculous. (Therefore, it does) not allow for modification without careful weighing.]

Jing Qian Xie Shui
Watery Discharge Prior to Menstruation

(Some) women have three days of watery discharge preceding their menstrual flow. People suppose (this to be due to) effulgent blood. Who would suspect spleen qi vacuity? The spleen governs the blood. When it is vacuous, it is no longer able to contain (the blood). Furthermore, as the spleen belongs to damp earth, when it is vacuous, earth becomes infirm. Conversely, when earth is infirm, dampness becomes more serious. If the spleen becomes *bu gu* or unconsolidated before the menstrual flow starts, the blood, which is governed by the spleen channel and is about to pour into the sea of blood, is overwhelmed by damp qi and, therefore, the menstrual flow is preceded by a watery discharge. The method of balancing menstruation does not consist of giving priority to the treatment of water but to that of blood. Or rather, it does not consist of giving priority to the treatment of blood but to the supplementation of qi. The reason is that, (on the one hand,) when qi is effulgent, blood will naturally be generated. On the other, when qi is effulgent, dampness will naturally be eliminated. Furthermore, when qi is effulgent, the menses will be restored to normal by itself. The formula to use is ***Jian Gu Tang*** (Fortify & Consolidate Decoction):

Radix Panacis Ginseng (*Ren Shen*), 5 *qian*
Sclerotium Poriae Cocoris (*Bai Fu Ling*), 3 *qian*
Rhizoma Atractylodis Macrocephalae (*Bai Zhu*), 1 *liang*, stir-fried with earth
Radix Morindae Officinalis (*Ba Ji*), 5 *qian*, soaked in salt water

Semen Coicis Lachryma-jobi (*Yi Yi Ren*), 3 *qian*, stir-fried

Decoct in water. Ten *ji* taken in succession (and) no water will be discharged before menstruation. This formula supplements the spleen qi to consolidate spleen blood. Thus blood is contained within qi and, as spleen qi gradually becomes exuberant, it recovers its ability to transport and transform dampness. When dampness is reduced to naught, menstruation will naturally be balanced and harmonized. How then can there be watery discharge before menstruation?

Jing Qian Da Bian Xia Xue Hemafecia Prior to Menstruation

(Some) women have blood in their stools one day before menstruation. People suppose this is a *xue beng* condition. Who would suspect the menses flowing into the large intestine? Since the menstrual flow takes a different route from that of the large intestine, how can it enter the large intestine? It should be understood that the *bao tai* ligation communicates with the heart above and the kidneys below. If the heart and kidneys fail to join or communicate, the blood of the *bao tai* can return to neither of them, and the qi of the heart and kidney channels stop coming to look after and restrain it, (thus) letting it (flow) free. Consequently, blood meanders into the large intestine instead of the small intestine. If treatment were to consist solely of stopping the blood in the large intestine, then, the more (done to) stop bleeding, the more (bleeding would be seen). If the qi of the triple burner should be hit and stirred, (blood) becomes more seriously disturbed and impossible to stop. This reckless wandering of the menstrual flow results from the loss of communication between the heart and the kidneys. If, however, no effort is made to put water and fire in a *ji ji* way but one merely treats the *bao tai*, how can blood return to the *jing*, since one has not provided the qi of the *bao tai* a place to which to return? Therefore, the heart and kidneys must be greatly supplemented to restore the connection between their qi. Then *bao tai* qi will no longer disperse, the blood in the large intestine will not move in a reckless way, and menstruation will be restored to normal. The formula to use is ***Shun Jing Liang An Tang*** (Normalize the Menses, Calm the Two Decoction):

Radix Angelicae Sinensis (*Dang Gui*), 5 *qian*, washed with wine
Radix Albus Paeoniae Lactiflorae (*Bai Shao*), 5 *qian*, stir-fried with wine
Radix Coquitus Rehmanniae (*Da Shu Di*), 5 *qian*, steamed 9 times
Fructus Corni Officinalis (*Shan Yu Rou*), 2 *qian*, steamed
Radix Panacis Ginseng (*Ren Shen*), 3 *qian*
Rhizoma Atractylodis Macrocephalae (*Bai Zhu*), 5 *qian*, stir-fried with earth
Tuber Ophiopogonis Japonicae (*Mai Dong*), 5 *qian*, cored
Herba Seu Flos Carbonisatus Schizonepetae Tenuifoliae (*Hei Jie Sui*), 2 *qian*
Radix Morindae Officinalis (*Ba Ji Rou*), 1 *qian*, soaked in salt water
Rhizoma Cimicifugae (*Sheng Ma*), 4 *fen*

Decoct in water and take. Two *ji* (and) the blood in the large intestine is stopped and the menstrual flow is led out from the anterior secret organ (*i.e.*, the vagina); 3 *ji* (and) the menstrual flow is stopped, (thus) also making conception possible. This formula greatly supplements the three channels of the heart, liver, and kidneys with no care for the *bao tai*. The reason why the *bao tai* now finds somewhere to which to return is that heart and kidney qi now communicate. When the heart and the kidney qi are vacuous, their qi separate. When they are sufficient, their qi unite with each other. Since the qi of the *bao tai* resigns itself to being governed by these two channels, how can it behave in a reckless way when the heart and kidneys are closely linked? It is understandable to supplement the heart and kidneys in case of loss of communication between them, but why is it necessary to simultaneously supplement liver/wood? It should be understood that the liver is the child of the kidneys and the mother of the heart. When the liver is supplemented, its qi travels to and fro between the heart and kidneys. It naturally goes up to conduct heart (qi) down to the kidneys and goes down to conduct the kidney (qi) up to the heart. It, (therefore,) serves as a go-between. This is an important method for restoring the interaction between the heart and the kidneys and its application is not limited to regulation of menstruation. Students should try to understand this deeply.

[Excessive blood in the stools, lack of *jing shen* (essence spirit or affect), and growing emaciation are surely due to spleen injury by enduring depression in turn due to unsoothed liver qi. An injured spleen failing to govern blood requires a different treatment (from the above). The formula to use (in that case) is *Bu Xue Tang* (Supplement the Blood Decoction): Radix Astragali Seu Hedysari (*Huang Qi*), 2 *liang*, half raw, half steamed; Radix Angelicae Sinensis (*Gui Shen*), 4 *qian*, washed with wine & char-fried; charred Radix Albus Paeoniae Lactiflorae, (*Hang Bai Shao*), 2 *qian*, scorched Rhizoma Atractylodis Macrocephalae (*Bai Zhu*), 5 *qian*, stir-fried with earth; Cortex Eucommiae Ulmoidis (*Du Zhong*), 2 *qian*, stir-fried till fibers are broken; charred Herba Seu Flos Schizonepetae Tenuifoliae (*Jing Jie*), 2 *qian*; Rhizoma Carbonisata Zingiberis (*Jiang Tan*), 2 *qian*. This preparation is taken with 1 *qian* of Rhizoma Carbonisata Guanzhong (*Guan Zhong Tan*). Four *ji* will surely effect a cure. After a cure, reduce (the amount of the preparation) to half and administer 2 more *ji*. Trespassing of blood into the large intestine invariably occasions blood in the stool during menstruation. At the initial stage, essence spirit usually remains normal in spite of this trespassing of the blood. But failure of the spleen to govern the blood must result in abnormal essence spirit. This should be distinguished.]

Lao Wei Nian Jing Shui Duan
Premature Menopause

The classic (*i.e.*, the *Nei Jing*) states: "(In) females, at 7 times 7 (or at around 49 years of age), the *tian gui* is exhausted." But there are (cases of) menopause under the age of seven times seven. People suppose (this to be due to) withered blood menstrual block (amenorrhea). Who would suspect depression of the heart, liver, and spleen qi? Suppose the blood were exhausted; how could life have been sustained in this world for long? This is an arbitrary presumption that some physicians give whenever they encounter menopause. (However, premature menopause) is not due to exhausted blood but (rather) to menstrual block. What's more, the menstruation is not blood but heavenly water or the *tian gui*. Originating in the kidneys, it is the essence of consummate yin (the kidneys), but possessed of the qi of consummate yang (the heart). Therefore, it is red like blood but it is, in fact, not blood. This accounts for its name, the *tian gui* or heavenly water. People nowadays regard the menstrual flow as blood, but this is an incorrect assumption, (in fact,) an unshakable assumption for 1,000 years. If it were blood, why should it be named menstrual flow (literally, *jing shui*, menstrual water) rather than menstrual blood (*jing xue*)? This name, *jing shui*, is derived from the belief that it comes from the kidneys and is transformed by the heavenly stem *gui*. Regrettably, people accept conventional ideas without giving profound consideration to their implications and look upon (the menstruate) as blood. It seems, however, that kidney water should be debilitated and dried up in the case of premature menopause. The reason why, I think, that it is (due to) depression of the heart, liver, and spleen qi is that the *generation* of kidney water, in fact, has nothing to do with the heart, liver, or spleen. Rather, it is the *transformation* of kidney water that is concerned with these three. Suppose there is no earth qi to sustain water from beneath. Then water floods over to extinguish fire, and kidney qi is unable to transform. Suppose there is no water qi to sustain fire from beneath. Then fire burns flaming to melt metal, and kidney qi can in no way be engendered. Suppose there is no metal qi to sustain wood from beneath. Then wood becomes wild (enough) to break earth, and kidney qi cannot take shape. If any one of the channels of the heart, liver, or spleen is depressed and its qi is consequently unable to enter the kidneys, then the qi of the kidneys will be depressed and become non-diffusive, let alone when the heart, liver, and spleen are all depressed. Even though it were really abundant and not really depleted, kidney qi would be in a predicament similar to a lump stuck in the throat (in which case, it is difficult to spit out what is taken in). If, in fact, kidney qi's root were vacuous, how could it get brimmingly full and be able to transform and discharge the menstrual flow? This is what is implied in the explanation of the classic that hyperactivity is harm.[5] This is why *jing bi* or menstrual block seems due to withered blood but, practically (speaking), it is not. The treatment must be to dissipate depression of the heart, liver, and spleen and to greatly supplement kidney water. In fact, to greatly supplement kidney water is to greatly supplement the qi of the heart, liver, and spleen. As a result, essence (will be full enough to) spill and the menses will recover its free flow by itself. The formula to use is ***Yi Jing Tang*** (Boost the Menses Decoction):

---

5 At first glance, the word hyperactivity seems inconsistent in this context, but, in fact, it is not. This passage focuses on an argument against ascription of premature menopause to withering of the blood, implying that repletion or superabundance is responsible.

Radix Coquitus Rehmanniae (*Da Shu Di*), 1 *liang*, steamed 9 times
Rhizoma Atractylodis Macrocephalae (*Bai Zhu*), 1 *liang*, stir-fried with earth
Radix Dioscoreae Oppositae (*Shan Yao*), 5 *qian*, stir-fried
Radix Angelicae Sinensis (*Dang Gui*), 5 *qian*, washed with wine
Radix Albus Paeoniae Lactiflorae (*Bai Shao*), 3 *qian*, stir-fried with wine
Semen Ziziphi Spinosae (*Sheng Zao Ren*), 3 *qian*, pounded
Cortex Radicis Moutan (*Dan Pi*), 2 *qian*
Radix Glehniae Littoralis (*Sha Shen*), 3 *qian*
Radix Bupleuri (*Chai Hu*), 1 *qian*
Cortex Eucommiae Ulmoidis (*Du Zhong*), 1 *qian*, char-fried
Radix Panacis Ginseng (*Ren Shen*), 2 *qian*

Decoct in water. Eight *ji* taken in succession (and) the menstruation will recover its free flow. Thirty *ji* (and) menstrual block will disappear making conception possible as well. This formula treats the channels of the heart, liver, spleen, and kidneys simultaneously. Its subtlety lies in not only supplementing but freeing the flow and not only dissipating but (also) opening. If only supplementation were applied, depression would not be opened but instead would generate fire. If only dissipating were employed, qi would become all the more debilitated and essence the more consumed. If attacking hardness prescriptions and hot, acrid ingredients were used, harm rather than good would be done.

Book 2

Nu Ke Gynecology (Continued)

Chapter 1

Ren Shen
Pregnancy

Ren Shen E Zu
Pregnancy Malign Blockage
(*i.e.*, Morning Sickness)

(Some) pregnant women suffer from nausea, retching, and vomiting with desire for sour (things) to quench their thirst but an aversion to any food in sight, fatigue, and somnolence. People all call this *ren shen e zu* or pregnancy malign blockage. Who would suspect extreme dryness of liver blood? Conception in women is based on effulgent kidney qi. Only when the kidneys are effulgent, can the *jing* essence be contained. However, once the kidneys have received the essence (from the male) and generated pregnancy, kidney water begins to grow the fetus (and becomes) too busy to moisten the five *zang*. The liver is the child of the kidneys and has to live on the qi of its mother every day to be soothed. Whenever it is in need of nourishing fluids, its qi will be pressing for them. As now kidney water is unable to meet this demand, the liver becomes more impetuous or temperamental. When the liver becomes impetuous, fire stirs with (liver qi) counterflow. Once liver qi counterflow occurs, problems such as retching, vomiting, and nausea arise. Retching and vomiting may not be too serious, but qi will inevitably be injured all the same. (And if) the qi is injured, liver blood will be all the more consumed. Physicians nowadays employ *Si Wu Tang* to treat the various gestational disorders just because that formula is capable of generating liver blood. Although it may not be wrong to supplement the liver to generate its blood, if the blood is generated without also making efforts to generate the qi, frequent retching cannot be conquered by a debilitated, weak spleen and stomach. And, as long as the qi is vacuous, blood will still not be easy to generate. Because of this, besides (ingredients) to level the liver and supplement blood, medicinals to fortify the spleen and open the stomach should be used to (help) generate yang qi. Qi is (thus) able to generate the blood and this is particularly helpful to the fetal qi.

The question may be asked, however, if one uses qi supplementing ingredients in the presence of qi counterflow, will this not promote the counterflow? It should be understood that, in terms of morning sickness, this counterflow is not very serious. What's more, this counterflow is caused by vacuity rather than evils. Counterflow due to evils is promoted (if qi is supplemented). But counterflow due to vacuity is rectified by supplementing the qi. Furthermore, because (in this formula) supplementation of qi is incorporated into supplementation of blood, yin is made abundant (enough) to restrain yang. Therefore, how can there be any worry about promoting counterflow? It is appropriate to use ***Shun Gan Yi Qi Tang*** (Normalize the Liver, Boost the Qi Decoction):

Radix Panacis Ginseng (*Ren Shen*), 1 *liang*
Radix Angelicae Sinensis (*Dang Gui*), 1 *liang*, washed with wine
Fructus Perillae Frutescentis (*Su Zi*), 1 *liang*, stir-fried & ground

Rhizoma Atractylodis Macrocephalae (*Bai Zhu*), 3 *qian*, stir-fried with earth
Sclerotium Poriae Cocoris (*Fu Ling*), 2 *qian*
Radix Coquitus Rehmanniae (*Shu Di*), 5 *qian*, steamed 9 times
Radix Albus Paeoniae Lactiflorae (*Bai Shao*), 3 *qian*, stir-fried with wine
Tuber Ophiopogonis Japonicae (*Mai Dong*), 3 *qian*, cored
Pericarpium Citri Reticulatae (*Chen Pi*), 3 *fen*
Fructus Seu Semen Amomi (*Sha Ren*), 1 piece, stir-fried & ground
Massa Medica Fermentata (*Shen Qu*), 1 *qian*, stir-fried

Decoct in water. One *ji* (and) mitigation is effected; a second *ji* (and) improvement is effected; a third *ji* (and) complete cure is effected. This formula levels the liver (resulting in) elimination of liver counterflow. It supplements the kidneys, putting an end to liver dryness. And it supplements qi, making it easy to generate the blood. For any fetal disorder (*tai bing*) with slight morning sickness, this formula can be prescribed and be effective without fail. It is extremely helpful for pregnant women, being even more effective than *Si Wu Tang*.

[It is suspected that 1 *liang* is mistaken for 1 *qian* for Fructus Perillae Frutescentis.]

Ren Shen Fu Zhong
Swelling & Edema in Pregnancy

(Some) women in the fifth month of pregnancy suffer from fatigued limbs, inability to taste food, and swelling gradually spreading from the feet to the whole body, including the head and face. People suppose (this is due to) damp qi. Who would suspect vacuity of spleen and lung qi? Although, during pregnancy the fetus is nourished according to a monthly (law)[1], (treatment) should, in practice, not be limited to the number of months and, in any case, spleen-fortifying and lung-supplementing should be used on general principle. The reasons are that, because the spleen controls blood while the lungs govern the qi and because the fetus cannot be nourished without blood or delivered without qi, blood can be made effulgent to nourish the fetus when the spleen is fortified. Whereas, qi is made effulgent to give birth to a child when the lungs are made clear. (Conversely,) when the lungs are debilitated, qi shrivels and when qi is shrivelled, no qi is transported to the skin. In addition, when the spleen is vacuous, blood becomes short, and when blood is short, no blood is transported to the limbs. Because of dual vacuity of qi and blood and dual dysfunction of the spleen and lungs, food is difficult to disperse and refined essence is no longer transformed. It follows, (therefore,) that qi and blood are bound to fall, incapable of uplifting, while damp evils take advantage of the empty place to accumulate and develop into a water swelling disease. Is this not caused by dual vacuity of spleen blood and lung qi? The treatment method should be to supplement spleen blood and lung qi. In this way, there is no need to dispel dampness, dampness cannot but depart. The formula to use is ***Jia Jian Bu Zhong Yi Qi Tang*** (Modified Supplement the Center, Boost the Qi Decoction):

Radix Panacis Ginseng (*Ren Shen*), 5 *qian*
Radix Astragali Seu Hedysari (*Huang Qi*), 3 *qian*, use raw
Radix Bupleuri (*Chai Hu*), 1 *qian*
Radix Glycyrrhizae (*Gan Cao*), 1 *fen*
Radix Angelicae Sinensis (*Dang Gui*), 3 *qian*, washed with wine

---

1 It is believed that the fetus receives nourishment in turn from the various viscera and bowels, or rather the channels and connecting vessels, in a monthly order and that it is better to treat fetal disorders in conformity with this law.

Rhizoma Atractylodis Macrocephalae (*Bai Zhu*), 5 *qian*, stir-fried with earth
Sclerotium Poriae Cocoris (*Fu Ling*), 1 *liang*
Rhizoma Cimicifugae (*Sheng Ma*), 3 *fen*
Pericarpium Citri Reticulatae (*Chen Pi*), 3 *fen*

Decoct in water. Four *ji* taken (and) cure is effected; 10 *ji* prevent relapse. As (this formula) was originally designed to upraise the qi of the spleen and lungs, *Bu Zhong Yi Qi Tang* seems to boost qi without supplementing the blood. However, because the blood cannot be generated without qi, supplementing qi is as good as generating blood. This issue becomes clear (when this formula is) compared with *Dang Gui Bu Xue Tang* in which Radix Astragali Seu Hedysari (*Huang Qi*) is introduced as the ruler. Furthermore, in cases where damp qi takes advantage of vacuity of the spleen and lungs to invade, it is not proper to greatly supplement blood for fear that too exuberant (righteous) yin should court (evil) yin. When (ingredients) which only supplement qi are used with dampness disinhibitors as assistants, qi ascends and water becomes particularly easy to dissipate. Consequently, the blood is generated. Why, however, is as much as 1 *liang* of Sclerotium Poriae Cocoris used? (In this case,) is not this dampness disinhibitor nearly made the ruler? Oh, well! If not this medicinal, what else should be made the ruler for a damp condition? What's more, together with medicinals to supplement qi, the inclusion of Sclerotium Poriae Cocoris in large amounts, though indeed aimed at percolating dampness, nonetheless serves the purpose of fortifying the spleen and clearing the lungs. Moreover, it is true that nearly all water disinhibitors are qi-consuming medicinals, but the combined use of Sclerotium Poriae Cocoris in considerable amounts with Radix Panacis Ginseng and Rhizoma Atractylodis Macrocephalae supplements more than it disinhibits. Therefore, its use in (large) amounts results in separating damp evils and this, (in turn,) results in supplementing qi and blood.

Ren Shen Shao Fu Teng
Lower Abdominal Pain in Pregnancy

Lower abdominal aching or pain during pregnancy and *tai dong bu an* or restless stirring of the fetus which seems to threaten abortion is thought merely (due to) weakness of the *dai mai*. Who would suspect spleen and kidney depletion? It is true that the *bao tai* is linked to the *dai mai*, but the *dai mai* is related to the spleen and kidneys. It is because of depleted and reduced spleen and kidney (function) that the *dai mai* becomes weak. Consequently, the *bao tai* has nothing to hold it (up). Furthermore, people's spleen and kidneys become depleted either because of serious food injury or because of excessive sexual intercourse. If the spleen and kidneys become depleted, the *dai mai*'s (situation) becomes urgent and the *bao tai*, therefore, exhibits signs of sagging. Since the *bao tai* ligation, however, has access to the heart and the kidneys but not to the spleen, it is understandable to supplement the kidneys. But why is it necessary to supplement the spleen? The spleen is *hou tian* or latter heaven; while the kidneys are *xian tian* or earlier heaven. The spleen without the qi of earlier heaven cannot transform. While the kidneys without the qi of latter heaven cannot generate. If one were to supplement the kidneys but not supplement the spleen, how can kidney essence be generated quickly? Because of this, supplementing the *hou tian* spleen is as good as supplementing the *xian tian* kidneys. (And,) supplementing the *xian tian* kidneys and the *hou tian* spleen is as good as consolidating the qi and blood of the *bao tai*. (Thus,) is it not necessary to supplement both the spleen and the kidneys? The formula to use is ***An Dian Er Tian Tang*** (Calm & Establish the Two Heavens Decoction):

Radix Panacis Ginseng (*Ren Shen*), 1 *liang*, stemless
Radix Coquitus Rehmanniae (*Shu Di*), 1 *liang*, steamed 9 times
Rhizoma Atractylodis Macrocephalae (*Bai Zhu*), 1 *liang*, stir-fried with earth
Radix Dioscoreae Oppositae (*Shan Yao*), 5 *qian*, stir-fried
Radix Praeparatus Glycyrrhizae (*Zhi Cao*), 1 *qian*
Fructus Corni Officinalis (*Shan Yu*), 5 *qian*, steamed, cored
Cortex Eucommiae Ulmoidis (*Du Zhong*), 3 *qian*, char-fried
Fructus Lycii Chinensis (*Gou Qi*), 2 *qian*
Semen Dolichoris Lablabis (*Bian Dou*), 5 *qian*, stir-fried, skinned

Decoct in water. One *ji* taken (and) pain is relieved; a second *ji* taken (and) the fetus becomes quiet. Because *tai dong* or stirring fetus is a spleen/kidney dual depletion condition, prompt rescue cannot be expected unless yin and yang supplementing medicinals, such as Radix Panacis Ginseng, Rhizoma Atractylodis Macrocephalae, and Radix Coquitus Rehmanniae, are used in large amounts. People nowadays usually dare not use, or use but a little, Radix Panacis Ginseng and Rhizoma Atractylodis Macrocephalae. Therefore, they rarely achieve effect though they wish to accomplish a feat. The subtlety of this formula lies just in employing (these medicinals) in large amounts.

[Radix Panacis Ginseng, 1 *liang*, can be replaced by Radix Codonopsis Pilosulae (*Dang Shen*). In default of Radix Codonopsis Pilosulae of good quality, tender Radix Astragali Seu Hedysari (*Huang Qi*) can (also) be substituted.]

Ren Shen Kou Gan Yan Teng
Dry Mouth & Sore Throat in Pregnancy

(Some) women in the third or fourth month of pregnancy commonly (experience) a dry mouth, parched tongue, and slight sore throat accompanied by an absence of fluids to moisten, and may even suffer from stirring of restless fetus. In serious cases, (there may be) bleeding like menstrual flow. People suppose (this is due to) extremely stirring or agitated fire. Who would suspect seriously depleted water? The fetus or *tai* is originally the product of combined essence and blood and is nourished according to a monthly (law or progression). The ancients used to assign the channels and connecting vessels (to each month's nourishment or development). Practically (speaking, however), kidney water is indispensable in nourishing (the fetus all the time). This is because, when kidney water is abundant, the fetus is calm. (But,) when kidney water is depleted, the fetus stirs and becomes agitated. Depleted kidney water, of course, has no means to stir the fetus (itself). It is stirring of the fire of the kidney channel that makes the fetus stir or become agitated. Nonetheless, in the last analysis, insufficiency of water underlies superabundance of fire. Therefore, when fire is flaming, the fetus invariably becomes agitated, but when water is supplemented, the fetus is naturally calmed. Here the *ji ji* approach is once again implied. Kidney water, however, cannot be generated quickly (by itself). Therefore, it is vital to enrich and supplement lung/metal. When metal is moistened, water is generated and afforded the pleasure of meeting with a spring. Once water finds its source and (is supplied by) a gushing spring, how can it be difficult to overwhelm fire? If a small amount of heat-clearing medicinals is added, the fetus will certainly be calmed. The formula to use is ***Run Zao An Tai Tang*** (Moisten Dryness, Calm the Fetus Decoction):

Radix Coquitus Rehmanniae (*Shu Di*), 1 *liang*, steamed 9 times
Radix Rehmanniae (*Sheng Di*), 3 *qian*, stir-fried with wine
Fructus Corni Officinalis (*Shan Yu Rou*), 5 *qian*, steamed
Tuber Ophiopogonis Japonicae (*Mai Dong*), 5 *qian*, cored
Fructus Schizandrae Chinensis (*Wu Wei*), 1 *qian*, stir-fried

Gelatinum Corii Asini (*E Jiao*), 2 *qian*, stir-fried with powdered clam shell
Radix Scutellariae Baicalensis (*Huang Qin*), 2 *qian*, stir-fried with wine
Herba Leonuri Heterophylli (*Yi Mu*), 2 *qian*

Decoct in water. Two *ji* taken (and) dryness is ended; 2 more *ji* taken (and) the fetus is calm. Ten *ji* taken in succession (and) the fetus will never stir. This formula is particularly capable of replenishing the essence of the kidneys and is, at the same time, able to supplement the lungs. Supplementation of the lungs, however, itself serves the purpose of supplementing the kidneys. In consequence, when the kidney channel is free from dryness, fire is no longer able to burn. Then how can the fetus be restless?

[This formula is perfectly miraculous. It offers an immediate cure. In no case should medicinals such as Radix Sophorae Subprostratae (*Shan Dou Geng*) or Rhizoma Belamcandae Chinensis (*She Gan*) be used because of sore throat. Nor is it acceptable due to excessive moisture to add Sclerotium Poriae Cocoris (*Yuan Ling*).]

Ren Shen Tu Xie Fu Teng
Vomiting, Diarrhea, & Abdominal Pain in Pregnancy

(Some) pregnant women suffer from vomiting and diarrhea, stirring fetus bordering on abortion, and unbearable abdominal pain too acute to be relieved. This is caused by extreme vacuity of the spleen and stomach. When spleen and stomach qi are vacuous, the *bao tai* becomes weak and there will certainly exist the danger of profuse (uterine) bleeding and miscarriage. What's worse, because of vomiting above and diarrhea below, the qi of the spleen and stomach are made even more vacuous. How can the *bao tai* be expected to be safe and secure? What then is the reason that, despite uterine pain, abortion does not occur? This is entirely due to consolidation of the kidney qi. The *bao tai* is linked to the kidneys and is associated with the heart. As long as kidney qi is *gu* or consolidated and is connected with the heart, the qi has free flow or access to the *bao tai*. This is why the *bao tai* threatens but does not miscarry. What's more, if kidney qi can manage to consolidate, yin fire will surely come and generate the spleen. (And, if) heart qi can manage to flow freely, heart fire will surely come to the aid of the stomach. The spleen and stomach may already be vacuous but have not yet expired. Therefore, the fetus stirs but has not (yet) aborted. Thus, is there any other choice but to give emergency aid to the spleen and stomach? However, since the spleen and stomach, though not yet expired, are already on the verge of expiration, it is difficult to generate them quickly if they alone are rescued. It is, (therefore,) proper to supplement, in addition, the fire of the heart and kidneys in order for them to (help) engender earth. When these two are brought into contact, the fetus will become consolidated and calm. The formula to use is ***Yuan Tu Gu Tai Tang*** (Support Earth, Consolidate the Fetus Decoction):

Radix Panacis Ginseng (*Ren Shen*), 1 *liang*
Rhizoma Atractylodis Macrocephalae (*Bai Zhu*), 2 *liang*, stir-fried with earth
Radix Dioscoreae Oppositae (*Shan Yao*), 1 *liang*, stir-fried
Cortex Cinnamomi (*Rou Gui*), 2 *qian*, sorted & ground
Radix Praeparatus Aconiti Carmichaeli (*Zhi Fu Zi*), 5 *fen*
Radix Dipsaci (*Xu Duan*), 3 *qian*
Cortex Eucommiae Ulmoidis (*Du Zhong*), 3 *qian*, char-fried
Fructus Corni Officinalis (*Shan Yu*), 1 *liang*, steamed, cored
Fructus Lycii Chinensis (*Gou Qi*), 3 *qian*
Semen Cuscutae (*Tu Si Zi*), 3 *qian*, stir-fried with wine

Fructus Seu Semen Amomi (*Sha Ren*), 3 pieces, stir-fried & ground
Radix Praeparatus Glycyrrhizae (*Zhi Gan Cao*), 1 *qian*

Decoct in water. One *ji* taken (and) diarrhea is stopped; a second *ji* taken (and) all other problems are cured. Eight tenths of this formula is allotted to salvaging spleen and stomach earth, while two tenths (is allotted) to the fire of the heart and kidneys. Is saving fire given less (priority) to saving earth because earth borders on expiration while fire is not as yet so debilitated? No. The explanation is that, when earth is about to collapse, it cannot be supported unless the dose is large; while debilitated fire can be assisted by even a small dose. Used in large quantities, hot ingredients, which are unlike warm, sweet ingredients, are sure to incur the danger of over-drying. What's more, since fetal stirring is due to debilitated earth rather than to weak fire, what is the point in utilizing too hot (medicinals)? Cortex Cinnamomi and Radix Praeparatus Aconiti Carmichaeli are (ordinarily) prohibited during pregnancy since they may typically injure the fetus. (Therefore,) how can they be used in large amounts? Slightly hot medicinals can be used only by the *qian*, while intensely hot ones only by the *fen*. These are used to conduct rather than to invigorate fire. This merits deliberate consideration.

Ren Shen Zi Xuan Xie Teng
Fetal Suspension with Lateral Costal Pain in Pregnancy

(Some) pregnant women are so overwhelmed by worry and depression that they have fetal stirring with oppression and pain in their lateral costal regions which (feel as tight) as a fully drawn bow-string. People know no more than that this is (so-called) fetal suspension disease (*zi xuan zhi bing*).[2] Who would suspect liver qi not flowing freely? The fetus half relies on kidney water for nourishment, but, without the assistance of liver blood, kidney water finds it difficult to persist. Therefore, in order to consolidate the fetus, kidney water must be enriched and the liver blood also must needs be taken into account. When liver qi is free from depression, liver qi is free from being blocked. Liver blood then surely will become effulgent (and) naturally able to irrigate the *bao tai*. (Thus, it is able) to join kidney water in sharing the burden of nourishing the fetus. If liver qi is blocked and obstructed due to worry and depression, as a result, the fetus loses blood nurturance and the kidneys find it difficult to fulfil their duty single-handed. How then can the fetus (be expected) not to rise in search of food? Depressed qi should be held responsible for this. Do not believe that it will be alright when medicinals to drain the fetus are employed on the assumption that the fetus can suspend itself by its own will. The appropriate treatment method is to open the depression and binding of the liver qi and supplement dried liver blood. Then the suspended fetus will automatically settle (back into place). The formula to use is ***Jie Yu Tang*** (Resolve Depression Decoction):

Radix Panacis Ginseng (*Ren Shen*), 1 *qian*
Rhizoma Atracylodis Macrocephalae (*Bai Zhu*), 5 *qian*, stir-fried with earth
Sclerotium Poriae Cocoris (*Bai Fu Ling*), 3 *qian*
Radix Angelicae Sinensis (*Dang Gui*), 1 *liang*, washed with wine
Radix Albus Paeoniae Lactiflorae (*Ba Shao*), 1 *liang*, stir-fried with wine
Fructus Citri Seu Ponciri (*Zhi Qiao*), 5 *fen*, stir-fried

2 Fetal suspension implies that the fetus has moved up too far under the ribs. It is not being carried down low enough in the abdomen.

Fructus Seu Semen Amomi (*Sha Ren*), 3 pieces, stir-fried & ground
Fructus Gardeniae Jasminoidis (*Shan Zhi Zi*), 3 *qian*, stir-fried
Herba Menthae (*Bo He*), 2 *qian*

Decoct in water. One *ji* taken (and) oppression and pain are relieved; a second *ji* taken (and) fetal suspension is settled; a third *ji* taken (and) a complete cure is effected. Administer several more *ji* with Fructus Gardeniae Jasminoidis deleted and relapse will be prevented. This is a divine formula for levelling the liver and resolving its depression. Once depression is opened, wood will no longer restrain earth, and, once the liver is level, fire will no longer stir recklessly. Because (this formula) is also composed of medicinals which fortify the spleen and open the stomach, water essence will naturally spread to every corner. Since the liver and kidneys are able to receive moisture, the fetus will naturally be rid of the affliction of dryness. Is there any need to worry that fetal suspension will not be cured?

[It is even better if 3-4 *qian* of Semen Coicis Lachryma-jobi (*Yi Yi Ren*) are added.]

Ren Shen Die Sun
Impact Injury in Pregnancy

(Some) pregnant women experience impact damage from falls and hence suffer from injured fetal origin (*shang tai yuan*) with abdominal pain threatening to induce imminent abortion. People know no more than that this is a disease resulting from external injury. Who would suspect that it is caused by an existing internal injury? So long as people have no other disease in the interior, the fetal origin is strong and consolidated. Even in case of fall, wrenching, or contusion, they are safe and sound. Only if the internal qi and blood have been depleted, can the fetus be disturbed by contusion or wrenching, however slight it be. If this is treated simply as an external injury due to contusion or wrenching, cure is nearly impossible, and there are cases where abortion is induced by (erroneous) treatment. Does this not require caution? It is necessary to greatly supplement the qi and blood and to use (only) a small amount of medicinals to remove stasis. Thus stasis will be dispersed and the fetus will become calm. In greatly supplementing qi and blood, if blood-supplementing medicinals are more than qi-supplementing ones, gain will be yielded without fail. The formula to use is ***Jiu Sun An Tai Tang*** (Rescue Damage, Calm the Fetus Decoction):

Radix Angelicae Sinensis (*Dang Gui*) 1 *liang*, washed with wine
Radix Albus Paeoniae Lactiflorae (*Ba Shao*), 3 *qian*, stir-fried with wine
Radix Rehmanniae (*Sheng Di*), 1 *liang*, stir-fried with wine
Rhizoma Atractylodis Macrocephalae (*Bai Zhu*), 5 *qian*, stir-fried with earth
Radix Praeparatus Glycyrrhizae (*Zhi Gan Cao*), 1 *qian*
Radix Panacis Ginseng (*Ren Shen*), 1 *qian*
Lignum Sappanis (*Su Mu*), 3 *qian*, pounded
Gummum Olibani (*Ru Xiang*), 1 *qian*, de-oiled
Myrrha (*Mo Yao*), 1 *qian*, de-oiled

Decoct in water. One *ji* taken (and) pain is relieved; a second *ji* taken, the tendency to abortion is thwarted. A third *ji* is unnecessary. The subtlety of this formula lies in its ability to remove stasis without injuring the fetus and to supplement qi and blood without causing congelation or stagnation. Therefore, while it is free of the risks attendant to flow-freeing and disinhibiting, it is able to heal the impact injury. Being beneficial without causing any harm, this is a formula that works wonders. What's more, it is a formula not only specifically effective for contusion and wrenching during pregnancy but also efficacious for such injuries (even in those) not pregnant.

[It is best to use ordinary Rhizoma Atractylodis Macrocephalae scorched-fried with earth, since it is capable of regulating the qi and moving the blood. *Yu Bai Zhu*[3] is too sweet to regulate the qi or move the blood. This is one (of the pieces) of knowledge required of a physician.]

Ren Shen Xiao Bian Xia Xue Bing Ming Tai Lou
Hematuria During Pregnancy, (also) Called Fetal Leakage

(Some) pregnant women frequently have blood in the urine with no fetal stirring and no abdominal pain. People suppose (this) to be fetal leakage or *tai lou* due to blood vacuity. Who would suspect qi vacuity failing to contain blood? The fetus is nourished by nothing but blood, but the blood nourishing the fetus must rely on the qi as its defender. When qi is vacuous and falls, the blood nourishing the fetus also falls with it. However, when the qi is vacuous and falls, if blood is not necessarily vacuous, seemingly, it ought not fall with the qi. It should be understood that qi is the defender of the blood and the blood relies on the qi to consolidate it. When qi is vacuous, blood has nothing on which to rely, and, without anything to rely upon, it will become dry and impetuous. This dryness and impetuosity then generates or gives rise to heat. When cold, blood is tranquil, but when hot, it is agitated and stirs. Once stirred, it must come out and cannot be stopped. How can it not flow down? If qi is not vacuous and the blood is hot, this

3 This is an undomesticated Atractylodes. In modern times, it is no longer available commercially. *Yu* is the shorthand name for *Yu Qian*, a county in Zhejiang Province.

then leads to *da beng* or great flooding, and, if this is not stopped, (it will eventually become) a small amount of *lou* or leakage. The appropriate treatment method is to supplement insufficient qi and drain superabundant fire. Thus bleeding is stopped automatically without stopping bleeding, (*i.e.*, without using *zhi xue* medicinals.) The formula to use is ***Zhu Qi Bu Lou Tang*** (Assist the Qi, Supplement the *Lou* Decoction):

Radix Panacis Ginseng (*Ren Shen*), 1 *liang*
Radix Albus Paeoniae Lactiflorae (*Bai Shao*), 5 *qian*, stir-fried with wine
Radix Scutellariae Baicalensis (*Huang Qin*), 3 *qian*, char-fried with wine
Radix Rehmanniae (*Sheng Di*), 3 *qian*, char-fried with wine
Herba Leonuri Heterophylli (*Yi Mu Cao*), 1 *qian*
Radix Dipsaci (*Xu Duan*), 2 *qian*
Radix Glycyrrhizae (*Gan Cao*), 1 *qian*

Decoct in water. One *ji* taken (and) bleeding is stopped; a second *ji* taken, and leakage is stopped. This formula uses Radix Panacis Ginseng to supplement yang qi and Radix Scutellariae Baicalensis to drain yin fire. When fire is drained, blood will be no longer hot and (thus becomes) disinclined to stir. When qi is made effulgent, blood will be afforded backing and there will be no (open) portals (from which) to leak. When qi and blood are both effulgent and in harmony, they naturally return to the channels and become calm in their own abodes. Then where is the trouble of leakage and spillage?

[It is admirable to use Radix Angelicae Sinensis to supplement blood for it is an aromatic and dry medicinal.]

Ren Shen Zi Ming
Fetal Crying in Pregnancy

(Some) women in the seventh or eighth month of pregnancy suddenly experience the fetus crying from within the abdomen (accompanied by) dull pain in the lumbar region. People suppose (this) to be due to fetal heat. Who would suspect that it is caused by qi vacuity? The appropriate treatment is to greatly supplement the qi, and the formula to use is ***Fu Qi Zhi Ti Tang*** (Support the Qi, Stop the Crying Decoction):

Radix Panacis Ginseng (*Ren Shen*), 1 *liang*
Radix Astragali Seu Hedysari (*Huang Qi*), 1 *liang*, use raw
Tuber Ophiopogonis Japonicae (*Mai Dong*), 1 *liang*, cored
Radix Angelicae Sinensis (*Dang Gui*), 5 *qian*, washed with wine
Exocarpium Citri Rubri (*Ju Hong*), 5 *fen*
Radix Glycyrrhizae (*Gan Cao*), 1 *qian*
Radix Trichosanthis Kirilowii (*Hua Fen*), 1 *qian*

Decoct in water. One *ji* taken (and) crying is brought to a pause; a second *ji* taken, crying stops once and for all. This formula uses Radix Panacis Ginseng, Radix Astragali Seu Hedysari, and Tuber Ophiopogonis Japonicae to supplement the lung qi. Once the lung qi is made effulgent, the qi of the uterus (also) becomes effulgent. Once the uterus qi is effulgent, how can the fetal qi in the uterus not breathe in step with its mother's qi?

[(In terms of) Radix Astragali Seu Hedysari, use the tender or *Nen Huang Qi*. Do not use the arrow or *Jian Qi*. *Jian Qi* is, in fact, the root of Medicago Sativa (*Mu Xu Geng*) produced north of Zhangjiakou.]

Ren Shen Yao Fu Teng Ke Han Zao Kuang Ji Zi Kuang
Fetal Mania, (*i.e.*), Lumbar & Abdominal Pain, Thirst, Sweating, & Mania in Pregnancy

(Some) women during pregnancy become thirsty, sweat (spontaneously), and drink cold water in great quantities and then suffer from vexation, agitation, mania, lumbar, and abdominal pain which eventually induces abortion. People all declare (this due to) extremely exuberant fire, but do they know in which channel this fire is so effulgent? It is the fire in the stomach that is flaming intensely and boils the water in the uterus. As a result, the water in the uterus is dried up and the fetus loses that which nourishes it. Thus is stirs and becomes restless. The stomach is the *shui gu zhi hai* or sea of water and grain and a channel abundant in qi and blood. The reason why it nourishes all the five viscera and six bowels is that every (living) thing arises from the earth. Only when earth qi is thick, do things begin to grow, and when earth qi is thin, things are doomed to death. However, earth qi can grow thick only on condition that fire qi comes to generate it. And the stomach is able to transform water and grain only on condition that fire is able to transform (it). If there is fire in the stomach, a favorable (situation) for generating earth, then why does exuberant fire do it harm instead? It should be understood that it is true that earth is difficult to generate without fire, but fire, if excessive, will dry up water. It is true that earth lives on as long as there is fire in it, but it is free from dryness only when there is (also) water. Suppose the fire in the stomach is over-effulgent. This will inevitably dry up kidney water. If earth becomes devoid of water, how can it spare any water to moisten the uterus when it has not enough to moisten even itself? When earth is burning extremely intensely, the blazing flames gain such momentum that they invade the heart and trespass against the *shen* or spirit. Once the fetus is (so) oppressed, how can it be prevented from sagging? This is just what is meant by the statement in the classic that, "Disease of the two yang expands to the heart and spleen." The treatment method must be to drain fire and enrich water. Once water qi is made effulgent, fire qi automatically becomes calm, and, when fire qi is calm, sweating, mania, agitation, and thirst are naturally eliminated. The formula to use is ***Xi Fen An Tai Tang*** (Quench the Conflagration, Calm the Fetus Decoction):

Radix Rehmanniae (*Sheng Di*), 1 *liang*, stir-fried with wine
Herba Artemisiae Apiaceae (*Qing Hao*), 5 *qian*
Rhizoma Atractylodis Macrocephalae (*Bai Zhu*), 5 *qian*, stir-fried with earth
Sclerotium Poriae Cocoris (*Fu Ling*), 3 *qian*
Radix Panacis Ginseng (*Ren Shen*), 3 *qian*
Rhizoma Anemarrhenae (*Zhi Mu*), 2 *qian*
Radix Trichosanthis Kirlowii (*Hua Fen*), 2 *qian*

Decoct in water. One *ji* taken (and) mania is alleviated a little; a second *ji* taken, mania is largely settled; a third *ji* taken, fire is resolved completely and the fetus is calm. This formula is a very heavy composition. In anticipation of (some) not daring to use it for fear patients cannot stand it, it is necessary to give some more assurance. When fire is overwhelming to such an extent in pregnancy, what means can extinguish it except (such) a large dose? And, unless fire is put out, mania cannot be cured and how can the fetus be calm? Furthermore, large though (the dosages) are in quantity, the ingredients are but medicinals to enrich water. They can do anything but harm; so there is no need to worry.

Ren Shen Guo Nu Duo Tai
Falling Fetus (Due to) Excessive Anger During Pregnancy

(Some) women invariably miscarry when the fetus has or has not yet taken shape. People all declare (this to be due to) debilitated qi and blood failing to consolidate the fetus. Who would suspect rashness and irascibility (causing) liver fire (and thus) great stirring and restlessness? The liver is responsible for storing the blood. When one is angry, it fails to store and, when it fails to store, the blood becomes difficult to consolidate. Although the liver belongs to wood, in wood is hidden a dragon-thunderous fire, or, in other words, *xiang huo* or ministerial fire. Ministerial fire is suited to tranquility but not disturbance. Given tranquility, it is calm, (but, when) stirred or agitated, it burns ragingly. What's more, the fire within wood is easy to stir but difficult to tranquilize. In one's life, there is not a single day without disturbance. And that means that there is not a single day when fire is not stirred. In violent anger, fire is all the more stirred and, when stirring fire becomes uncontrollable, furious flames soar. Far from being able to generate qi or nourish the fetus, it consumes the qi and injures essence. Once essence is damaged, the fetus has nothing to nourish it and this cannot but end in abortion. This is just what is meant by the statement in the classic that, "Small fire generates qi; vigorous fire eats qi." To stop this, the appropriate treatment method is, (therefore,) to level the fire within the liver and disinhibit the qi of the lumbus and navel. Once qi is made to generate the blood and the blood to clear the fire, cure will be realized soon. The formula to use is ***Li Qi Xie Huo Tang*** (Disinhibit the Qi, Drain the Fire Decoction):

Radix Panacis Ginseng (*Ren Shen*), 3 *qian*

Rhizoma Atractylodis Macrocephalae (*Bai Zhu*), 1 *liang*, stir-fried with earth
Radix Glycyrrhizae (*Gan Cao*), 1 *qian*
Radix Coquitus Rehmanniae (*Shu Di*), 5 *qian*, steamed 9 times
Radix Angelicae Sinensis (*Dang Gui*), 3 *qian*, washed with wine
Radix Albus Paeoniae Lactiflorae (*Bai Shao*), 5 *qian*, stir-fried with wine
Semen Euryalis Ferocis (*Qian Shi*), 3 *qian*, stir-fried
Radix Scutellariae Baicalensis (*Huang Qin*), 2 *qian*, stir-fried with wine

Decoct in water. Sixty *ji* taken (and) abortion is prevented. This formula, though entitled qi-disinhibiting, in effect, supplements the qi. If, however, fire-draining ingredients were not added to (these) qi-supplementing (medicinals), then qi might become effulgent and fire would remain restless. Inevitably (this) would do qi harm instead of good. For this reason, Radix Scutellariae Baicalensis is added to the qi-supplementing (ingredients) in order to drain fire. Besides, there are Radix Coquitus Rehmanniae, Radix Angelicae Sinensis, and Radix Albus Paeoniae Lactiflorae to enrich the liver to invigorate the governance of water. Thus, blood is free from dryness and qi is brought into harmony, while angry qi is appeased and fire gets calm of itself. (In that event,) qi is relieved of inhibition without fail and without needing to use qi-disinhibitors. In short, (this formula) is never employed but that disinhibition is achieved.[4]

[In treating rashness and irascibility, use of liver-soothing medicinals is out of the question during pregnancy. The classic states: "(It is) fetal disease which leads to disease of the mother and, when the fetus is calm, the mother's disease is automati-

4 There is a pun here in Chinese which, unfortunately, cannot be adequately rendered in English.

cally cured." For that reason, gestational diseases are usually treated by supplementing the qi, nurturing the blood, and calming the fetus as the key. (If this is followed,) tens of thousands of diseases will naturally be cured.]

Chapter 2

Xiao Chan
Small Birth, (*i.e.*, Miscarriage)

Xing Fang Xiao Chan
Miscarriage (Due to) Sexual Intercourse

Miscarriage with incessant uterine bleeding caused by sexual intercourse in pregnant women is supposedly due to extreme fire stirring. Who would suspect that it is due to qi desertion? The profuse uterine bleeding originates from qi vacuity, whereas exuberant fire originates from water depletion. When kidney water is depleted, the source of generating qi becomes exhausted. With the source exhausted, how can qi (be expected) not to desert? This kind of stirring fire is the *biao* or branch; while qi desertion is the *ben* or root. The classic states: "Treat disease by tracing its root." Once the root is consolidated, the branch will take care of itself. If stopping bleeding alone is taken as the key without promptly consolidating the qi, qi will disperse and cannot return soon. Then how can bleeding be stopped? If essence is not greatly supplemented, water, which has become exhausted, is not able to grow quickly, while fire rages (even) more intensely. I have never seen anyone effect rescue by attending to the end instead of focusing on the root. The formula to use is *Gu Qi Tian Jing Tang* (Consolidate the Qi, Replenish the Essence Decoction):

Radix Panacis Ginseng (*Ren Shen*), 1 *liang*
Radix Astragali Seu Hedysari (*Huang Qi*), 1 *liang*, use raw
Rhizoma Atractylodis Macrocephalae (*Bai Zhu*), 5 *qian*, stir-fried with earth
Radix Coquitus Rehmanniae (*Da Shu Di*), 1 *liang*, steamed 9 times
Radix Angelicae Sinensis (*Dang Gui*), 5 *qian*, washed with wine
Radix Pseudoginseng (*San Qi*), 3 *qian*, ground fine, mixed in (after decocting the other ingredients)
Herba Seu Flos Schizonepetae Tenuifoliae (*Jie Sui*), 2 *qian*, char-fried

Decoct in water. One *ji* taken (and) bleeding is stopped; a second *ji* taken (and) the body is out of danger; a fourth *ji* taken, complete cure is effected. The subtlety of this formula lies in its supplementing qi and essence without (specifically) clearing fire. What accounts for its singular miraculous effect is that the various ingredients, which are warm and moistening, are (nonetheless) capable of eliminating intense heat. Because this heat is vacuity (heat), supplementing the qi by itself is capable of containing blood; while supplementing the essence is by itself capable of stopping bleeding. (This is because this formula) aims at the root.

[In most cases, miscarriage with profuse (uterine) bleeding is caused by sexual intercourse. In cases above 40 years of age, Radix Panacis Ginseng and Radix Astragali Seu Hedysari should be doubled in amount but Radix Coquitus Rehmanniae should be reduced to half. This is because qi is vacuous and fire is debilitated (in such cases). Otherwise, more often than not, qi will be made to desert irretrievably. In pregnancy, one should try to control their sexual desire and refrain from sexual intercourse. Take care and do not embark on the risky path.]

Die Shan Xiao Chan
Miscarriage (Due to) Wrenching & Contusion

(Some) pregnant women experience falls, contusion, or wrenching and subsequently suffer from miscarriage with bleeding of purple clots and clouding (of their senses) and faintness. All people declare (this to be due) to trouble caused by blood stasis. Who would suspect detriment of the *xue shi* or blood chamber? The blood chamber is connected with the uterus as the lips are to the teeth. When the uterus is injured, the blood chamber is damaged. With the lips gone, the teeth are (exposed to) cold. This is of necessity so. However, injury of the uterus causing bleeding is superficial, while detriment of the blood chamber causing bleeding is deep-seated. Superficial injury gives pain in the abdomen, whereas deep-seated injury causes faintness in the heart. Similar impact injuries may cause miscarriage or they may not. Their treatment, therefore, should not be the same. If there is no miscarriage but the fetus is *bu an* or not calm, it is proper to attend to the fetus and it is not permissible to eliminate blood without warrant. If there is miscarriage with enormously profuse bleeding, it is proper to dissipate stasis but it is not permissible to inflict new injury to the qi. After the fetus has aborted and the blood has deserted, the blood chamber is vacuous and empty and what is left is but the qi. If this qi were to be damaged in addition, (who) would dare guarantee against the worry of qi desertion? The classic states: "Blood is the *ying*, qi is the *wei*." If the *wei* or defense is *bu gu* or unconsolidated, the *ying*, with nothing to support it, cannot remain calm. Therefore, (in order) to generate blood, it is necessary to supplement qi. When new blood is generated, static blood will be dispersed automatically. The formula to use is ***Li Qi San Yu Tang*** (Regulate the Qi, Dissipate Stasis Decoction):

Radix Panacis Ginseng (*Ren Shen*), 1 *liang*

Radix Astragali Seu Hedysari (*Huang Qi*), 1 *liang*, use raw
Radix Angelicae Sinensis (*Dang Gui*), 5 *qian*, washed with wine
Sclerotium Poriae Cocoris (*Fu Ling*), 3 *qian*
Flos Carthami Tinctorii (*Hong Hua*), 1 *qian*
Cortex Radicis Moutan (*Dan Pi*), 3 *qian*
Rhizoma Carbonisata Zingiberis (*Jiang Tan*), 5 *qian*

Decoct in water. One *ji* taken (and) bleeding is stopped; a second *ji* taken, clouding and faintness are eliminated; a third *ji* taken, complete recuperation is effected. This formula uses Radix Panacis Ginseng and Radix Astragali Seu Hedysari to supplement the qi. Once qi is made effulgent, blood is contained. Radix Angelicae Sinensis and Cortex Radicis Moutan are used to generate the blood. Once blood is generated, stasis will find it difficult to remain. Flos Carthami Tinctorii and Rhizoma Carbonisata Zingiberis are used to quicken the blood. Once blood is quickened, faintness is relieved. Sclerotium Poriae Cocoris is used to disinhibit water. Once water is disinhibited, blood will find it easy to return to the channels.

[For the non-miscarriage case, it is proper to add Cortex Eucommiae Ulmoides (*Du Zhong*), char-fried, 1 *qian*, and Radix Dipsaci (*Xu Duan*), char-fried, 1 *qian*. For the miscarriage case, administer the above formula unchanged. In case of incessant *xue beng*, add charred Rhizoma Guanzhong (*Guan Zhong*) , 3 *qian*. In case of blood block cardiac faintness (*xue bi xin yun*), add charred Rhizoma Corydalis Yanhusuo (*Yan Hu Suo*), 1 *qian*.]

Da Bian Gan Jie Xiao Chan
Miscarriage with Dry, Knotted Stools

(Some) pregnant women suffer from thirst, vexation and agitation, tongue sores, swollen, cracked lips, dry, knotted stools, constipation (lasting for) several days, and subsequently have abdominal pain and even miscarriage. People all declare (this is due to) fire/heat of the large intestine. Who would suspect hot blood burning the fetus? Blood, as a fetus-nourishing substance, benefits the fetus when it is warm but injures it when it is excessively hot. If (blood) remains hot for long and burns, the child in the uterus will suffer such torment as if in boiling water, (so much so) that it becomes difficult for (the child) to survive. It has no other choice but to move out and run down in order to escape the flaming oppression. How then can abortion of the fetus be avoided? Because it nourishes the fetus, blood is necessarily consumed and grows vacuous (during pregnancy). Blood is yin. When blood becomes vacuous, yang must become hyperactive. Hyperactivity (of yang) does harm. Furthermore, blood is transformed from yin/water. Because blood, which has to nourish the fetus every day, demands supplies urgently, whereas fire is burning ragingly, yin/water cannot be generated quickly enough for the transformation of blood. As a result, yin becomes vacuous and fire is stirred. Because (now) yin is full of nothing but fire and blood is full of nothing but fire, these two fires join each other to burn and oppress the fetus so that the fetus drops. The appropriate treatment methods are to clear fire from the uterus and to supplement the essence in the kidneys. Then everything will be alright. It may be questioned why the uterus should be the (main) concern, since the fetus has aborted, and why water should be greatly supplemented, since it is blood that fails to nourish the fetus. It should be understood that, when fire stirs to such an extreme extent that it results in abortion, the uterus is entirely filled with masses of fire qi. This fire is a vacuity fire. Replete fire allows for drainage, but vacuity fire requires clearing by way of supplementation. In this way, vacuity fire is easy to dissipate and true fire will be generated. If cool, clearing ingredients are used exclusively to downbear fire without any regard to whether the uterus is vacuous or replete, cold qi will certainly be made to oppress in a menacing way. Thus, the vital qi is left in dire meagerness in the stomach. The stomach, which is the second yang, nourishes and provides supplies for the five viscera. If stomach yang stops being generated, what else can transform the refined essence to generate yin/water? Few cases (treated in this erroneous way) can avoid changing into consumptive disease. The formula to use is ***Jia Jian Si Wu Tang*** (Modified Four Ingredient Decoction):

Radix Coquitus Rehmanniae (*Shu Di*), 5 *qian*, steamed 9 times
Radix Albus Paeoniae Lactiflorae (*Bai Shao*), 3 *qian*, use raw
Radix Angelicae Sinensis (*Dang Gui*), 1 *liang*, washed with wine
Rhizoma Ligustici Wallichii (*Chuan Xiong*), 1 *qian*
Fructus Gardeniae Jasminoidis (*Shan Zhi Zi*), 1 *qian*, stir-fried
Fructus Corni Officinalis (*Shan Yu*), 2 *qian*, steamed & cored
Radix Dioscoreae Oppositae (*Shan Yao*), 3 *qian*, stir-fried
Cortex Radicis Moutan (*Dan Pi*), 3 *qian*, stir-fried

Decoct in water. Four or five *ji* taken (and) a cure is effected. Because Cortex Radicis Moutan is, by nature, extremely capable of cooling the blood, the danger of congealing yin that it may induce when employed in postpartum cases must be guarded against. Take care!

[It is still better if 2 *qian* of thin Radix Astragali Seu Hedysari (*Tiao Qin*) are added to this formula.]

Wei Han Fu Teng Xiao Chan
Aversion to Cold & Abdominal Pain with Miscarriage

(Some) pregnant women experience aversion to cold and abdominal pain which results in miscarriage. About this, people know (no more than) excessive cold in the lower portion. Who would suspect qi vacuity failing to contain the fetus? Human beings are given birth to and nurtured by fire, but they cannot be replenished without qi. When qi is effulgent, fire is effulgent. When qi is debilitated, fire is debilitated. It is because of receiving true fire from its parents prenatally or *xian tian* that the human fetus is conceived. It is this earlier heaven true fire (*xian tian zhi zhen huo*) which gives rise to the development of the earlier heaven true qi (*xian tian zhi zhen qi*). Because of this, the fetus develops from and is contained by the qi. When qi is effulgent, the fetus is firm. When qi is debilitated, the fetus falls. As the fetus grows day by day, so the qi day by day becomes debilitated. Thus how can there be calm and not falling? What's more, if cold qi happens to invade from the outside, internal fire qi becomes (even) more feeble. Enfeebled fire qi has no means to nurture (the fetus) for long. Therefore, the fetus cannot help but fall. If medicinals, such as Radix Panacis Ginseng (*Ren Shen*) and Rhizoma Desiccata Zingiberis (*Gan Jiang*) had been administered in time to supplement qi and dispel cold when abdominal pain first began, the pain could have been relieved and the fetus calmed. Regrettably, however, the physician, (blindly) adhering to the medicinal contraindications of pregnancy, dares not employ these medicinals only unless abortion actually happens. (But) by now, there is left but an iota of qi. There are no other means but to rescue qi without delay. The formula to use is ***Huang Qi Bu Qi Tang*** (Astragalus Supplement Qi Decoction):

Radix Astragali Seu Hedysari (*Huang Qi*), 2 *liang*, use raw
Cortex Cinnamomi (*Rou Gui*), 5 *fen*, coarse bark sorted out, ground
Radix Angelicae Sinensis (*Dang Gui*), 1 *liang*, washed with wine

Decoct in water. Five *ji* taken (and) a cure is effected. If the case is ascribed to cold, and hot, acrid (ingredients) are accordingly used in large amounts without (medicinals) to (also) supplement qi and blood, such a formula, being too dry and hot, would probably cause yang collapse and turn the case critical.

Da Nu Xiao Chan
Miscarriage (Due to) Great Anger

Following great or intense anger, (some) pregnant women suddenly contract abdominal pain and vomit blood. Subsequently, they miscarry after which the abdominal pain persists. People suppose (this to be due to) unappeased angry fire of the liver. Who would suspect that it is caused by blood failing to return to the channels? The liver stores the blood, but during intense anger, blood cannot be stored. As a result, blood should be lost but abortion (*duo tai*, literally falling fetus) should not occur. Then why does abortion follow loss of blood? It should be understood that, because the liver is the most impetuous of all (the organs) by nature, if the blood's gate is unshut, blood will rush directly into the uterus. The *bao tai* ligation passes between the heart and the kidneys. When liver blood comes surging, the passageway connecting the heart and the kidneys is unavoidably cut. As a result of this broken passageway, the uterus can no longer be nurtured by water and fire. Therefore, the fetus falls. (However,) once the fetus has fallen, why does abdominal pain continue as before? The reason is that the heart and the kidneys have not yet joined. They incline but have no means to resume their connection. (This) painfully hurts the liver qi which is rejected when it comes to the heart and is denied reception when it comes to the kidneys. Therefore, blood is not yet tranquilized and pain still persists. The appropriate treatment method is to conduct liver blood back to the liver again. Then abdominal pain will disappear by itself. Simply conducting liver blood without levelling liver qi, however, cannot easily succeed in regulating qi counterflow or lead counterflow blood back (to the liver). The formula to use is ***Yin Qi Gui Xue Tang*** (Conduct the Qi, Return the Blood Decoction):

Radix Albus Paeoniae Lactiflorae (*Bai Shao*), 5 *qian*, stir-fried with wine
Radix Angelicae Sinensis (*Dang Gui*), 5 *qian*, washed with wine
Rhizoma Atractylodis Macrocephalae (*Bai Zhu*), 3 *qian*, stir-fried with earth
Radix Glycyrrhizae (*Gan Cao*), 1 *qian*
Herba Seu Flos Carbonisatus Schizonepetae Tenuifoliae (*Hei Jie Sui*), 3 *qian*
Cortex Radicis Moutan (*Dan Pi*), 3 *qian*
Rhizoma Carbonisata Zingiberis (*Jiang Tan*), 5 *fen*
Rhizoma Cyperi Rotundi (*Xiang Fu*), 5 *fen*, stir-fried with wine
Tuber Ophiopogonis Japonicae (*Ma Dong*), 3 *qian*, cored
Tuber Curcumae (*Yu Jin*), 1 *qian*, stir-fried with vinegar

Decoct in water and take. Though entitled qi-conducting, this formula, in fact, is capable of conducting blood. To conduct blood, however, it is to necessary to conduct qi. As qi returns to the liver, blood returns to the liver too. When both qi and blood return, abdominal pain will cease of itself.

Chapter 3

Nan Chan
Difficult Delivery

Xue Xu Nan Chan
Blood Vacuity Difficult Delivery

(Some) pregnant women, after several days of abdominal pain still are not able to give birth. People all declare (this to be due to) qi vacuity and weak strength failing to send the child out of the birth gate. Who would suspect inability of the child to turn over owing to blood vacuity, gluey stagnation, and absence of blood in the uterus? The fetus is originated from the essence of the kidneys, but it is nourished by the blood of the five viscera and six bowels. Because of this, when blood is effulgent, the child is easy to deliver. When blood is debilitated, the child becomes difficult to deliver. For this reason, in the days before delivery, it is proper to administer blood-supplementing ingredients. Because the blood is not generated quickly by means of blood-supplementing (alone), it (also) requires supplementation of qi to (help) generate it. However, only supplementing the qi is not appropriate, for (in that case) yang will probably become over-effulgent, while blood remains, nonetheless, insufficient. (If qi) prevails (over blood), the harm is invariably (the presence of) only upraising without downbearing and this results in difficult delivery. To guard against this tendency while still slight, the only choice is to supplement qi and blood simultaneously. When they both are made effulgent, qi is enabled to push (the fetus), while blood is sufficient to ferry it (out). Being in an ocean, (the fetus,) of course, has no difficulty turning itself. Where is the worry about gluey stagnation? The formula to use is ***Song Zi Dan*** (Send Off the Child Elixir):

Radix Astragali Seu Hedysari (*Sheng Huang Qi*), 1 *liang*
Radix Angelicae Sinensis (*Dang Gui*), 1 *liang*, washed with wine
Tuber Ophiopogonis Japonicae (*Mai Dong*), 1 *liang*, cored
Radix Coquitus Rehmanniae (*Shu Di*), 5 *qian*, steamed 9 times
Rhizoma Ligustici Wallichii (*Chuan Xiong*), 3 *qian*

Decoct in water. Two *ji* taken (and) the child will be delivered without the trouble of transverse presentation. This is a formula to supplement both qi and blood. (In it,) blood-supplementing ingredients are comparatively greater in amount than qi-supplementing ingredients except for one, Radix Astragali Seu Hedysari, which is used to supplement qi. While the rest in the formula are all ingredients to supplement the blood. When blood is effulgent, qi is afforded that which nourishes it. When qi is generated, blood is afforded that which it relies upon. Since the *bao tai* is moistened and lubricated, delivery will naturally be easy. This is likened to a stranded boat in a shallow place. It is impossible for it to move even though it is drawn by a great deal of manpower. But suddenly a spring flood happens to come! The boat will get ready to move by itself. Once there is a favorable wind blowing in addition, it will of course move swiftly under full sail.

Jiao Gu Bu Kai Nan Chan
Difficult Delivery (Due to) the Joined Bones Not Opening

(Some) pregnant women's babies are already at the *chan men* or birth gate but the child is unable to descend. This is a critical juncture of life and death. People suppose (this is due to) earlier than necessary broken placenta and dried up water failing to furnish slipperiness. Who would suspect that it is caused by non-movement of the joined bones? Over the birth gate there are two bones, which are named the joined bones.[1] They are connected closely. Before labor, the bones are so closely fit as to show not a single seam like the cloak of the sky. But towards delivery, these bones come apart as the door is opened. In females, the muscles of the baby gate (*er men*) grow obliquely and skin grows transversely so that the gate can be widened or narrowed, enlarged or made smaller. If it were not for the connection between these joined bones, the baby gate would certainly be open wide enough for the hand to go in and fetch out the placenta. These joined bones form the lower part of the baby gate, something in females like the bar in a lock. If these bones were not shut, the intestines would drop out at once, but, if they do not open, the child is difficult to deliver. However, it is the qi and blood which govern the opening and closing of these bones. If the blood is effulgent but the qi is debilitated, the child is able to descend but the baby gate does not open. Whereas, if the qi is effulgent but the blood is debilitated, the gate opens but it is difficult for the child to descend. It follows, (therefore,) that it is qi that opens these joined bones, while it is blood that turns the child. To have an easy delivery, the only choice is to greatly supplement (both) qi and blood. However, it is easy to shut but

---

1 This is a reference to the pubic bones.

difficult to open these joined bones. In most cases, non-movement of these joined bones during labor results from indulgence during pregnancy in sexual intercourse with the draining of too much essence. Once essence is drained, qi and blood lose the root of their generation and transformation and become seriously depleted. When qi and blood are depleted, nothing is transported to moisten the baby gate and, as a result, the joined bones stick to each other, unable to open. In order for these joined bones to move, it is necessary to employ bone-moving medicinals in addition to (ingredients) for supplementing the qi and blood. With these two kinds of medicinals combined in treatment, there will certainly be no trouble in opening (these bones). And, without taking the trouble of hastening delivery, the child will come forth rapidly by itself and mother and child will be both safe and sound. The formula to use is ***Jiang Zi Tang*** (Downbearing the Child Decoction):

Radix Angelicae Sinensis (*Dang Gui*), 1 *liang*
Radix Panacis Ginseng (*Ren Shen*), 5 *qian*
Rhizoma Ligustici Wallichii (*Chuan Xiong*), 5 *qian*
Flos Carthami Tinctorii (*Hong Hua*), 1 *qian*
Radix Cyathulae (*Chuan Niu Xi*), 3 *qian*
Ramulus Xylosmae Racemosae (*Zuo Mu Zhi*), 1 *liang*

Decoct in water and take. After one *ji* is taken, the baby gate is sure to give a loud crack. Then the joined bones separate and with that the child is delivered. This formula uses Radix Panacis Ginseng to supplement the qi, Rhizoma Ligustici Wallichii and Radix Angelicae Sinensis to supplement blood, Flos Carthami Tinctorii to quicken blood, Radix Cyathulae to downbear, and Ramulus Xylosmae Racemosae to open the pass and separate the bones. These four flavors (*i.e.*, the first four ingredients) cooperate in a harmonious way and what accounts for (this formula's) miraculous effect is the incorporation of separation within supplementation. Even though simply using Ramulus Xylosmae Racemosae may succeed in separating the bones anyhow without supplementing qi and blood, (in that case,) it will most likely be difficult to close bones) after (thus) separating (them). This is (also) very likely to induce the trouble of windstroke in the lower part (of the body). Therefore, it is less wonderful than the above formula which is able not only to separate but to close. Besides, in no case can Ramulus Xylosmae Racemosae (alone) be administered to open the gate before the child has approached it. But administering *Jiang Zi Tang* does no harm since it is able to supplement qi and blood. If ever Ramulus Xylosmae Racemosae is used alone, it must be administered (only) when (the child) has come to the gate.

Jiao Shou Xian Xia Nan Chan
Hand or Foot Comes Down First
Difficult Delivery, (*i.e.*, Breach Presentation)

In the process of giving birth, some women may be unable to deliver the child because it has its foot or hand out first. People suppose (this is due to) transverse or inverted presentation. This is an extremely critical case. Who would suspect that it is caused by dual vacuity of qi and blood? If the birthing woman's qi and blood is sufficient, the fetus is surely in a normal (position). If her qi and blood is depleted, the fetus is surely in a counterflow, (*i.e.*, abnormal position). Normal (position) makes delivery easy, while counterflow or abnormal (position) makes it difficult. If qi and blood are depleted, the mother must be weak and so must the child in the womb. Because it is so weak and flaccid, the child is not able to turn head down. Therefore, it has to have its hand or foot come out first. At this point, instantly needle the hand or foot of the child and it must withdraw away from the pain. To adjust its position as an emergence aid, administer promptly ***Zhuan Tian Tang*** (Turning Heaven Decoction):

Radix Panacis Ginseng (*Ren Shen*), 2 *liang*
Radix Angelicae Sinensis (*Dang Gui*), 2 *liang*, washed with wine
Rhizoma Ligustici Wallichii (*Chuan Xiong*), 1 *liang*
Radix Cyathulae (*Chuan Niu Xi*), 3 *qian*
Rhizoma Cimicifugae (*Sheng Ma*), 4 *fen*
Radix Praeparatus Aconiti Carmichaeli (*Fu Zi*), 1 *fen*

Decoct in water and take. One *ji* taken (and) the child is turned around; 2 more *ji* taken, (and the child) will naturally be delivered in a normal way. One of the subtleties of this formula lies in its using Radix Panacis Ginseng to supplement qi depletion and Rhizoma Ligustici Wallichii and Radix Angelicae Sinensis to supplement blood depletion. This is known to everyone. But the subtlety of using Rhizoma Cimicifugae besides Radix Cyathulae and Radix Praeparatus Aconiti Carmichaeli is probably seldom recognized. When the body of the child is already slanting, it is difficult to turn the head unless upraisers are employed. However, it is (still) difficult to downbear the body in the course of its turning unless (such) down-moving (ingredients) are used. Besides the combined use of Rhizoma Cimicifugae and Radix Cyathulae, Radix Praeparatus Aconiti Carmichaeli is used so that each and every channel is reached and so that qi and blood can be accelerated (thus) to hasten birth.

[After administration of 3 *ji* and needling the child's hand or foot, should the child still be unable to turn its body, needle the birthing woman at *He Gu* (LI 4) and the child will be delivered. Do not, in any event, put in the hand to probe and fetch the child out. This jeopardizes the lives of both the mother and the child. Do not do that!]

Qi Ni Nan Chan
Qi Counterflow Difficult Delivery

(Some) women fail to deliver the child after several days of labor and administration of various birth-hastening medicinals are of no avail. People suppose (this is due to) difficult movement of the joined bones. Who would suspect that it is due to qi counterflow and stagnation? It is true that non-movement of the joined bones can lead to difficult delivery, but that is responsible only for failing to deliver a child when its head has already come to the birth gate. (In that case,) the choice is naturally to employ the bone-moving formula. If the child's head has not yet come to the birth gate, what is most likely responsible is not non-movement of the joined bones but qi counterflow and stagnation which make it difficult for the child to turn its body around. If the joined bones were made to separate (by using the above formula erroneously), the baby gate would open wide and the child would descend with its head not yet turned down. This would inevitably lead to extraordinary transmuted patterns. For that reason, it is absolutely important not to open the baby gate unscrupulously. In childbirth, on the whole, it is improper to sit on straw too early.[2] If its head has not yet turned downward, there will still be a long time before the child will be delivered. If the birthing woman is made to sit on straw unduly early, she will become full of fear and apprehension when she has wait so long for the child to come out. Fear makes the spirit timid and timidity in turn makes the qi descend without the ability to ascend. Since qi does not ascend, the upper burner will be blocked, (thus) resulting in qi counterflow. When qi counter-

---

2 In old China, in many places women were made to sit on straw or a straw mat during birthing in order to keep clean. Hence, sitting on straw is equivalent to giving birth.

flow arises above, the upper burner surely becomes distended and full, making it more difficult for qi to move. Since qi is held up somewhere between the upper and the lower, simply hastening birth without disinhibiting qi only makes qi counterflow more serious and puts the fetus in a tighter blockage. The treatment method is to exclusively disinhibit the qi. Thus the child is enabled to turn round and come down by itself. The formula to use is ***Shu Qi San*** (Soothe the Qi Powder):

Radix Panacis Ginseng (*Ren Shen*), 1 *liang*
Radix Angelicae Sinensis (*Dang Gui*) 1 *liang*, washed with wine
Rhizoma Ligustici Wallichii (*Chuan Xiong*), 5 *qian*
Radix Albus Paeoniae Lactiflorae (*Bai Shao*), 5 *qian*, stir-fried with wine
Ramulus Perillae Frutescentis (*Zi Su Geng*), 3 *qian*
Radix Achyranthis Bidentatae (*Niu Xi*), 2 *qian*
Pericarpium Citri Reticulatae (*Chen Pi*), 1 *qian*
Radix Bupleuri (*Chai Hu*), 8 *fen*
Bulbus Allii Fistulosi (*Cong Bai*), seven *cun* long

Decoct in water and take. One *ji* (and) qi counterflow is rectified and the child will be delivered. This formula, though a qi-disinhibiting formula, actually supplements the qi. This qi counterflow is caused by qi vacuity because qi vacuity leads to susceptibility to fear. Once qi is supplemented, susceptibility to fear disappears and with it qi counterflow is settled without notice. Then why go to the trouble of moving the joined bones?

Zi Si Chan Men Nan Chan
Child Dead at the Birth Gate
Difficult Delivery

(Some) women have been in labor for three or four days, but, with the child already at the birth gate, the joined bones still refuse to open. Because it is unable to come out, the child dies. Although the mother survives, if the administration of bone-moving medicinals proves of no avail, she, too, faces the danger of death. The very reason that the mother is, luckily, not (yet) dead is none other than the death of the child and the dropping of the *bao tai*. The mother and child are subsequently separated and the mother's qi, which is already recovered, does not share the expiration of the child's qi. At this point, treatment should be only to rescue the mother without care for the child. However, the dead child lying at the birth gate blocks the lower opening of that gate, (thus) threatening the mother's life. Therefore, it is proper to employ a child pushing-conveying method of supplementing blood to generate water and supplementing qi to generate blood. When the qi and blood (of the mother) are both made effulgent, the dead child will come out and the mother's life will be saved. If child-downbearing (medicinals) alone are used to descend the child, it is most likely that the child will not be brought forth but that the mother's qi will first desert. This is not a good rescuing method. I have treated such cases personally, and the formula that I have often used, ***Jiu Mu Dan*** (Rescue the Mother Elixir), has saved many lives. Therefore it is given below.

Radix Panacis Ginseng (*Ren Shen*), 1 *liang*
Radix Angelicae Sinensis (*Dang Gui*), 2 *liang*, washed with wine
Rhizoma Ligustici Wallichii (*Chuan Xiong*), 1 *liang*
Herba Leonuri Heterophylli (*Yi Mu Cao*), 1 *liang*

Halloysitum (*Chi Shi Zhi*), 1 *qian*
Herba Seu Flos Schizonepetae Tenuifoliae (*Jie Sui*), 3 *qian*, char-fried

Decoct in water and take. One *ji* will bring forth the dead child. This formula uses Rhizoma Ligustici Wallichii and Radix Angelicae Sinensis to supplement the blood and Radix Panacis Ginseng to supplement the qi. When both qi and blood are effulgent, with qi able to push and blood able to convey, either ascension or descension can be executed. What's more, Herba Leonuri Heterophylli is good at bringing forth the dead child and Halloysitum is able to downbear blood stasis. Therefore, all will pour out at once without even slight obstruction or stagnation.

Zi Si Fu Zhong Nan Chan
Dead Child Within the Abdomen Difficult Delivery

(Some) women have been in labor for six or seven days, but, with the placenta already broken, the child fails to make its appearance. People suppose (this is a case of) difficult delivery. Who would suspect the child has died within the abdomen? It is easy to make a diagnosis if the child is dead at the baby gate, but it is difficult to determine if the child is dead within the abdomen. At the birth gate, the live child must be able to stretch and contract its head. (Whereas,) a dead child is still and remains so even when pushed by the hand. If alive, the child is sure to retreat if its hair is lightly touched by the hand. Therefore, (the diagnosis) is said to be easy. (But,) if the child is dead within the abdomen, what can help to determine this? There are, however, practical ways to determine this. In all cases of death within the abdomen, the mother, if savable, must not have any soot-black qi in her face. This indicates that the child is dead but that the mother's qi is not dead. If difficult to save, the mother will have soot-black qi in her face. This indicates that both the child is dead and the absence of life mechanism (*sheng ji*) in the mother. Following this to determine life and death, (one) will never be mistaken. In case of known death within the abdomen, use of medicinals to downbear (the child) is not allowed, for this is a dangerous way. The use of forcibly draining is also a dangerous way. Once labor has carried on for six or seven days, the mother's qi must be exhausted, no longer able to stand any kind of forcible treatment. If ever a forcible method is used to drive the dead child out, it is most likely that the mother will die with the dropping of the child. Still it is necessary to supplement the mother. Once her qi and blood are made effulgent, the dead child will drop by itself. The formula to use is ***Liao Er San*** (Treat the Baby Powder):

Radix Panacis Ginseng (*Ren Shen*), 1 *liang*
Radix Angelicae Sinensis (*Dang Gui*), 2 *liang*, washed with wine
Radix Cyathulae (*Chuan Niu Xi*), 5 *qian*
Gummum Olibani (*Ru Xiang*), 2 *qian*, de-oiled
Rhizoma Dysosmae Versipellis (*Gui Jiu*), 3 *qian*, water-ground

Decoct in water. One *ji* taken, the dead child is brought forth and the mother is saved. Without exception, it is not until it has turned its head downward that the child is delivered. If the child fails to turn its head downward, which is due to qi and blood vacuity of the mother, and the physician uses birth-hastening medicinals with the result that these consume the child's qi and blood, the child's qi will not enjoy free-reaching and the child will consequently be suffocated to death. Such a charlatan is virtually a murderer. For that reason, in the treatment of difficult delivery, birth-hastening medicinals are absolutely prohibited (and) supplementation of the qi and blood to strengthen the mother is the only proper treatment.

This may save countless lives of children. This formula is (designed) to rescue the mother with a dead child. Nevertheless, it greatly supplements qi and blood since it aims at rescuing the root. It should be understood that to rescue the root is as good as hastening birth.

[It is a subtle point) not to use Cortex Magnoliae Officinalis (*Hou Po*) to bring forth the dead fetus. There once was a case of a birthing woman with a black facial complexion and green-blue tongue who was administered medicinals to supplement her qi as well as to nurture and quicken the blood. The mother and the child were both saved, a lucky case of (one) in ten thousand.]

Chapter 4

Zheng Chan
Normal Delivery

Zheng Chan Bao Yi Bu Xia
Normal Delivery (but) the Placenta Does Not Descend

After the child is born, (some) women's placenta may remain stagnant within the abdomen and does not descend even (after) two or three days. (There is also) vexation of the heart, agitation of mind, and liability to clouding and dizziness. People suppose (this is due to) the pedicle of the placenta failing to come off. Who would suspect dry, withered blood adhering (the placenta) to the inside of the abdomen? Seeing that the placenta does not descend, people are usually full of worry and apprehension, fearing that (the placenta) might surge (up) to the heart producing signs of death. However, is it (really) possible for the placenta to surge up into the heart? When the placenta does not descend, static blood most probably moves with difficulty. Thus, blood dizziness well may be induced. The appropriate treatment is still to greatly supplement the qi and blood. When blood is generated to convey the placenta, the placenta will naturally be moistened and become slippery. Moisture and slipperiness make (its) descension easy. When qi is generated to assist the blood,

blood will naturally be generated rapidly, making it far easier to hasten the descension of the placenta. The formula to use is *Song Bao Tang* (Deliver the Uterus Decoction):

Radix Angelicae Sinensis (*Dang Gui*), 2 *liang*, washed with wine
Rhizoma Ligustici Wallichii (*Chuan Xiong*), 5 *qian*
Herba Leonuri Heterophylli (*Yi Mu Cao*), 1 *liang*
Gummum Olibani (*Ru Xiang*), 1 *liang*, not de-oiled
Myrrha (*Mo Yao*), 1 *liang*, not de-oiled
Herba Seu Flos Schizonepetae Tenuifoliae (*Jie Sui*), 3 *qian*, char-fried
Secretio Moschi Moschiferi (*She Xiang*), 5 *li*, ground, take separately

Decoct in water and take. Immediate precipitation will be effected. This formula uses Rhizoma Ligustici Wallichii and Radix Angelicae Sinensis to supplement the qi and blood, Herba Seu Flos Schizonepetae Tenuifoliae to conduct the blood back to the channels, and Herba Leonuri Heterophylli, Myrrha, and other medicinals to expel stasis and downbear the placenta. Once new blood is generated, old blood is impossible to remain. When qi becomes effulgent and ascends, static turbidity will naturally descend. How can there be affliction of retention and stagnation then? The placenta is what wraps the fetus. It is attached to both the child and to the mother. Its refusal to follow the child out during birthing shows that the child is not reliable. Therefore, it lingers (behind) in the abdomen as if it had filial compassion towards its mother. Although the abdomen of the mother has been delivered of the child, the pedicle (of the placenta) has not yet broken off (its) relation with the (mother's) qi. Therefore, (the placenta,) though on the verge of coming off, is reluctant to do so. In some cases, (the placenta) may be retained for six or seven days but it does not putrefy. The reason is simply that it still maintains life qi. It is obvious that a placenta retained in the abdomen cannot kill a person and that it will drop by itself when supplementation is applied. It may be questioned why the placenta should drop because of supplementation, since it is still possessed of life qi and should, therefore, get firmer and stronger with the supplementation of qi and blood. It should be understood that supplementation benefits the child before it is delivered but the mother after it is born. When the child benefits, the qi of the placenta becomes adhesive. When the mother benefits, the qi of the placenta deserts. There is a qi barrier or gate (*qi guan*) within the *bao tai*. When it is open, both (mother and child) are united. When it is shut, both are separated. For that reason, when qi and blood are greatly supplemented, the placenta will descend instead (of becoming more firmly attached).

Five or six days after the child is delivered, (some) women still have the placenta retained in their abdomen. Although one hundred means are tried, it refuses to drop but (yet) there are no signs of clouding, dizziness, vexation, or agitation. People suppose (this is due to) adhesion of static blood. Who would suspect vacuous qi being unable to push and convey? If there were static blood in the abdomen, it could not help making trouble, invariably causing dizziness. But, in this case, there is no trouble (and) blood proves already clean. With clean blood, clear qi is supposed to ascend, while turbid qi to descend. (But,) because the placenta is retained, clear qi does not downbear and has difficulty ascending. Therefore, turbid qi floats upward and is difficult to downbear. With turbid qi ascending, however, there ought to occur vexation and agitation. But, in this case, they do not. This is because neither clear nor turbid qi is able to ascend. However, if qi is supplemented, will not turbid qi be made to ascend? It should be understood that it is an invariable law that the clear ascends, while the turbid descends. There is never such an occasion when the clear ascends and the turbid also ascends. If clear and turbid qi are separated by supplementing the qi, (it is because) the clear is uplifted for the purpose of downbearing the turbid. The formula to use is ***Bu Zhong Yi Qi Tang*** (Supplement the Center, Boost the Qi Decoction):

Radix Panacis Ginseng (*Ren Shen*), 3 *qian*
Radix Astragali Seu Hedysari (*Sheng Huang Qi*), 1 *liang*
Radix Bupleuri (*Chai Hu*), 3 *fen*
Radix Praeparatus Glycyrrhizae (*Zhi Gan Cao*), 1 *fen*
Radix Angelicae Sinensis (*Dang Gui*), 5 *qian*
Rhizoma Atractylodis Macrocephalae (*Bai Zhu*), 5 *fen*, stir-fried with earth
Rhizoma Cimicifugae (*Sheng Ma*), 3 *fen*
Pericarpium Citri Reticulatae (*Chen Pi*), 2 *fen*
Semen Raphani Sativi (*Lai Fu Zi*), 5 *fen*, stir-fried & ground

Decoct in water and take. One *ji* taken (and) the placenta drops by itself. *Bu Zhong Yi Qi Tang* is a formula to raise qi rather than to push and convey it. Then why is it able to downbear the placenta so quickly? It is because the clear qi does not ascend that the turbid qi does not descend. When qi is raised, the clear ascends, while the turbid descends. With the descent of turbid qi, what is retained in the abdomen will, without fail, also descend. Therefore, it is needless to apply the pushing-conveying method. What's more, the inclusion of several *fen* of Semen Raphani Sativi is capable of regulating turbid qi so that the two kinds (of qi) will not interfere with each other. Because of this, the effect is wonderful.

Zheng Chan Qi Xu Xue Yun
Normal Delivery (but) Qi Vacuity, Blood Dizziness

Immediately following delivery, (some) women suddenly have dark eyes and flowery vision, retching, nausea, desire to vomit, and absence of governance in the heart or wandering *shen* spirit and *hun* as if walking amidst the clouds in the sky.[1] People suppose (this to be due to) trouble of malign blood surging into the heart. Who would suspect that it is due to qi vacuity bordering on desertion? In a recently birthed woman, all her blood must have poured out, the blood chamber must be empty and vacuous, and only a tiny amount of qi is left. If the woman had a vacuity of yang qi and was, (therefore,) unable to generate blood in the past, the blood in her heart has been consumed in nurturing the fetus. With the delivery of the child, this has further run out. Now the heart is left with no blood to nourish it, and the tiny amount of qi is what it relies on to secure it. What's worse, this qi is also now vacuous and about to desert. (Therefore,) the remnants of blood are unable to return to the channels (and thus) give rise to blood dizziness. The treatment method must be to greatly supplement the qi and blood, and it is absolutely improper to treat merely blood dizziness. It may be questioned that, if hot, blood will be helped to surge up with still greater momentum if blood is supplemented, since hot blood upsurging is the very cause of blood dizziness. It should be understood, (however,) that old blood will not disperse unless new blood is generated. To supplement the blood to generate blood is as good as quickening the blood to dispel old blood. However, blood, a tangible substance, is difficult to generate quickly, but qi, an intangible substance, is easy to generate quickly. (Because of

---

1 The *hun* is the so-called ethereal soul which resides in the liver.

that,) it is easier to supplement the qi in order to generate the blood than to supplement blood (alone). The formula to use is ***Bu Qi Jie Yun Tang*** (Supplement the Qi, Resolve Dizziness Decoction):

Radix Panacis Ginseng (*Ren Shen*), 1 *liang*
Radix Astragali Seu Hedysari (*Sheng Huang Qi*), 1 *liang*
Radix Angelicae Sinensis (*Dang Gui*), 1 *liang*, not washed with wine
Herba Seu Flos Carbonisatus Schizonepetae Tenuifoliae (*Hei Jie Sui*), 3 *qian*
Rhizoma Carbonisata Zingiberis (*Jiang Tan*), 1 *qian*

Decoct in water and take. One *ji* (taken), dizziness is relieved; a second *ji* (taken), the heart is stabilized; a third *ji* (taken), blood is generated; a fourth *ji* (taken), blood is effulgent and dizziness will never recur. This is a divine formula for resolving dizziness. It uses Radix Panacis Ginseng and Radix Astragali Seu Hedysari to supplement the qi in order that invigorated qi may generate the blood. Radix Angelicae Sinensis (is used) to supplement the blood in order that effulgent blood may nourish the qi. Once both qi and blood become effulgent, the heart will become stabilized by itself. It (also) uses charred Herba Seu Flos Schizonepetae Tenuifoliae to conduct blood back to the channels and charred Rhizoma Zingiberis to move stasis and conduct yang. Once static blood is gone, righteous blood will come back. Thus dizziness is resolved automatically without needing to resolve it (by using anti-dizziness medicinals symptomatically). How miraculous it is that a formula composed of but five ingredients is so wonderfully effective!

Zheng Chan Xue Yun Bu Yu
Normal Delivery (but) Blood Dizziness (&) Loss of Speech

As soon as the child has been delivered, (some) women have clouding and dizziness with loss of speech. This is (due to) dual desertion of qi and blood. This is (usually classified) among the unsavable (cases), but, if the method of rescue is appropriate, survival is not an impossibility. At the critical juncture, puncture promptly the midpoint between the eyebrows with a silver needle. When blood is let out, speech will be recovered. After that, decoct and pour down (the throat) 1 *liang* of Radix Panacis Ginseng (*Ren Shen*) and resurrection will be brought without fail. Life can also be brought back by pouring down (the throat) a bowl of a decoction named *Dang Gui Bu Xue Tang* (*Dang Gui* Supplement the Blood Decoction) composed of 2 *liang* of Radix Astragali Seu Hedysari (*Huang Qi*) and 1 *liang* of Radix Angelicae Sinensis (*Dang Gui*). Do not, by any means, add Radix Praeparatus Aconiti Carmichaeli (*Fu Zi*) without reason to either of these two formulas. Unlike Radix Panacis Ginseng, Radix Angelicae Sinensis, and Radix Astragali Seu Hedysari which come straight to the rescue of the expiring qi and blood and concentrate these and do not dissipate (them), Radix Praeparatus Aconiti Carmichaeli is able to reach each and every channel and spurs qi and blood medicinals to wander rather than keep to their position. Therefore, they cannot fasten on the uterus.

Generally speaking, clouding and dizziness in birthing in women are the kind of clouding and dizziness caused by a vacuous blood chamber with nothing to nourish the heart. The tongue is the sprout of the heart. Once the heart is without governance, how can the tongue utter voice? The midpoint between the eyebrows has access to the brain above and the tongue below. Whereas its ligation links with the heart. When (this area) is needled, both the brain and the tongue are freed and the clear qi of the heart ascends. Thus static blood naturally descends. After that, decoct and pour down (the throat) medicinals capable of supplementing qi and generating blood, such as Radix Panacis Ginseng, Radix Astragali Seu Hedysari, and Radix Angelicae Sinensis, and qi and blood will meet each other. How then can death possibly come? Simple administration of Radix Panacis Ginseng, Radix Astragali Seu Hedysari, and Radix Angelicae Sinesis may be able to avert death in some cases, but it is less wonderful than preceded by needling the midpoint between the eyebrows. People are acquainted only with the method of moxaing the midpoint between the eyebrows, but they do not know that needling excels this. Moxibustion is a slow method, while acupuncture is a quick method. It is difficult for (such) a slow (method) to rescue expiration, but it is easy for a quick (method) to bring back life. This is just what is meant by, "The quick treats the branch, while the slow treats the root."[2]

Zheng Chan Bai Xue Gong Xin Yun Kuang
Normal Delivery (but) Vanquished Blood Attacks the Heart (Causing) Dizziness (&) Mania

Two or three days after delivery, (some) women suffer from

---

[2] Normally, this line is translated, "In acute (conditions) treat the branch; in chronic (conditions) treat the root." However, in Chinese, the words for acute and quick and for chronic and slow are the same. Since Chinese grammar is very open-ended and since, in this context, the usual translation of this aphorism makes no sense, we have translated this saying differently than usual in this instance.

fever, retention of lochia, vanquished blood attacking the heart, manic ravings and shoutings, and, in serious cases, a desire to run about but hesitation in movement. People suppose (this is due to) trouble caused by evil heat in the stomach. Who would suspect that it is due to blood vacuity failing to nurture the heart? After delivery, because the blood has all gone with the fetus, the blood chamber becomes vacuous and empty. None of the viscera and bowels have any blood for nourishment and only in the heart is there a tiny amount of blood left to protect the heart sovereign. Because the viscera and bowels have nothing for nourishment, they are all inclined to turn to the heart for supplies. As premier of the heart sovereign, the *xin bao* or pericardium intercepts their qi and does not allow them to enter the heart so that calmness and tranquility of the heart spirit is ensured. Thus, the heart is protected entirely by the strength of the pericardium. If the pericardium is also vacuous and unable to serve as shelter for the heart, the qi of the various *zang* and *fu* will directly enter the heart to share heart blood. The pericardium is now in an urgent situation, unable either to look after its sovereign internally or to resist the (pressing) masses externally. It then raises its cries, giving signs bordering on mania and eccentricity and displaying a helpless desperation. Therefore, this disease shows evidence of heat, but, practically (speaking,) it is not a hot (disease). The treatment method must be to greatly supplement the blood in the heart in order for the viscera and bowels to share in its nourishment and to prevent them from harassing the heart anymore. Thus the heart will become composed and the pericardium quiet. The formula to use is ***An Xin Tang*** (Calm the Heart Decoction):

Radix Angelicae Sinensis (*Dang Gui*), 2 *liang*
Rhizoma Ligustici Wallichii (*Chuan Xiong*), 1 *liang*
Radix Rehmanniae (*Sheng Di*), 5 *qian*, stir-fried
Cortex Radicis Moutan (*Dan Pi*), 5 *qian*, stir-fried

Pollen Typhae (*Sheng Pu Huang*), 2 *qian*
Folium Nelumbinis Nuciferae (*Gan He Ye*), 1 leaf, as conductor

Decoct in water and take. One *ji* (taken,) mania is settled and the lochia is discharged as well. This formula uses Rhizoma Ligustici Wallichii and Radix Angelicae Sinensis to nurture the blood. But why are Radix Rehmanniae and Cortex Radicis Moutan added to cool the blood? This seems inappropriate in a postpartum case. It should be understood, (however,) that it is the attack of vacuity heat that causes the lochia to rush upon the heart. Cooling in combination with supplementation does no harm. What's more, with the help of Folium Nelumbinis Nuciferae, (they) free all seven portals and lead evil out, doing more than (just) preventing (evil) from doing harm to the heart internally. In addition, Pollen Typhae is used to assist in decomposing the lochia. Although this formula can be used to settle mania temporarily, it should not be used too often lest it incur trouble. Be cautious and discreet.

[After taking these medicinals and mania is settled, it is proper to take *Jia Wei Sheng Hua Tang* (Added Flavors Generate & Transform Decoction): Radix Angelicae Sinensis (*Dang Gui*), washed with wine, 1 *liang*, 1 *qian*; Rhizoma Ligustici Wallichii (*Chuan Xiong*), 3 *qian*; Semen Pruni Persicae (*Tao Ren*), ground, 1.5 *qian*; Herba Seu Flos Schizonepetae Tenuifoliae (*Jing Jie Sui*), char-fried, 1 *qian*; Cortex Radicis Moutan (*Dan Pi*), 1.5 *qian*. Best to take 4 *ji*.]

Zheng Chan Chang Xia
Normal Delivery (but) Intestinal Prolapse

Prolapse of the intestines in the birthing woman is, likewise, a critical condition. People suppose it to be due to non-closure of the *er men* or baby gate. Who would suspect vacuous and fallen qi failing to withdraw (the intestine)? In case of qi vacuity and falling, it is naturally proper to use up-raisers to lift the qi. However, because, in the newly delivered woman, there most likely exists static blood in the abdomen, if qi is raised, static blood might be brought up with it to soar into the upper (part of the body). This would cause the trouble of surging up into the heart which is likely to cause extraordinary transmuted patterns. Therefore, qi-raising cannot be carried out in a big way. Since this is so, what method can be adopted to treat (the qi) when qi has fallen? Generally speaking, qi falls because qi is vacuous. If it is merely supplemented, qi will become effulgent and the intestine will rise by itself. However, (only) a small amount of qi-supplementing medicinals will not be able to make the qi strong enough. Quantity, (in this case,) must count for much. Then yang will become effulgent and great in strength, and there will be no possibility that (the intestine) descends but will not ascend. The formula to use is ***Bu Qin Sheng Chang Yin*** (Supplement the Qi, Lift the Intestine Drink):

Radix Panacis Ginseng (*Ren Shen*), 1 *liang*, stem removed
Radix Astragali Seu Hedysari (*Sheng Huang Qi*), 1 *liang*
Radix Angelicae Sinensis (*Dang Gui*), 1 *liang*, washed with wine
Rhizoma Atractylodis Macrocephalae (*Bai Zhu*), 5 *qian*, stir-fried with earth
Rhizoma Ligustici Wallichii (*Chaun Xiong*), 3 *qian*, washed with wine
Rhizoma Cimicifugae (*Sheng Ma*), 1 *fen*

Decoct in water and take. One *ji* (taken, and) the intestine is lifted up. This formula solely supplements the qi without intestine-lifting (medicinals). Even the employment of 1 *fen* of Rhizoma Cimicifugae is (designed) merely to conduct and upbear qi. In terms of the use of Rhizoma Cimicifugae, a small amount lifts the qi, while a large amount raises the blood. This cannot be ignored.

Another formula uses 49 seeds of Semen Ricini Communis (*Bi Ma Ren*) which are pounded and applied on the vertex as an up-raiser. As soon as the intestine is lifted, they must be washed off, since long retention may induce vomiting of blood. This is an alternative method to up-bear the intestine.

Chapter 5

Chan Hou Postpartum (Disorders)

Chan Hou Shao Fu Tong Postpartum Lower Abdominal Pain

After delivery, (some) women have lower abdominal aching and pain. (If) severe, it may lead to binding and the formation of a mass, in which case, pressure makes the pain worse. People suppose this to be due to child's pillow pain or *er zhen zhi teng*. Who would suspect this trouble is caused by static blood? What is called the child's pillow was defined by our predecessors as that which the fetus pillows its head upon. (However,) if there is no pain when the fetus is pillowing (its head during gestation), how can one believe that pain arises owing to freedom from such pillowing after delivery of the fetus? It is obvious that this pain is not due to the (so-called) child's pillow. But then, what is the cause? It is caused by static blood which, not yet dispersed, binds into lumps. This condition is usually seen in strong women whose blood is superabundant rather than insufficient. (Therefore,) it would seem proper to use blood-cracking medicinals. When blood is quickened, stasis is naturally eliminated. Whereas, when blood binds, stasis causes trouble. But, if blood is vanquished instead of supplemented, though static blood is dispersed, consumption and depletion cannot be avoided. A better way is to incorporate the method of dispelling stasis into that of supplementing the blood. Thus stasis is dispersed completely, while qi and blood suffer no consumption. The formula to use is ***San Jie Ding Tong Tang*** (Scatter Binding, Settle Pain Decoction):

Radix Angelicae Sinensis (*Dang Gui*), 1 *liang*, washed with wine
Rhizoma Ligustici Wallichii (*Chuan Xiong*), 5 *qian*, washed with wine
Cortex Radicis Moutan (*Dan Pi*), 2 *qian*, stir-fried
Herba Leonuri Heterophylli (*Yi Mu Cao*), 3 *qian*
Herba Seu Flos Carbonisatus Schizonepetae Tenuifoliae (*Hei Jie Sui*), 2 *qian*
Gummum Olibani (*Ru Xiang*), 1 *qian*, de-oiled
Fructus Crataegi (*Shan Zha*), 10 pieces, char-fried
Semen Pruni Persicae (*Tao Ren*), 7 pieces, skinned and tip-nipped after soaking, stir-fried, & ground

Decoct in water. One *ji* taken, pain is relieved and cure is effected. A second *ji* is needless. This formula incorporates stasis-dispelling within blood-supplementing and is able to disperse clots while generating the blood. Its subtlety lies in stopping pain without specifically attacking it. People nowadays tend to use such medicinals as Rhizoma Corydalis Yanhusuo (*Yan Hu*), Lignum Sappanis (*Su Mu*), Pollen Typhae (*Pu Huang*), and Feces Trogopterori Seu Pteromi (*Ling Zhi*) to transform clots whenever they meet child's pillow. Their practice is beneath comment.

Postpartum lower abdominal pain in women which is relieved by pressure is also supposed to be pain due to child's pillow. Who would suspect that it is caused by blood vacuity? After delivery, too much blood is lost and the blood chamber is empty and vacuous. (In that case,) it is quite natural for abdominal pain to occur, and nine out of ten women suffer from it. This pain, however, is divided into two types: *xu* and *shi*, or vacuity and repletion. This distinction must not fail to be made. If (the pain is like that of) dry husks touching the body, it is vacuity pain rather than repletion pain. Generally speaking, vacuity pain is better treated by supplementation and this is especially the case with postpartum vacuity pain. Blood vacuity pain should only be treated with blood-supplementing medicinals. However, blood supplements are usually medicinals which moisten and lubricate and they may well interfere with the large intestine. In terms of postpartum blood vacuity, however, the intestines are usually dry. Therefore, moistening and lubricating are just what are desired. What kind of interference can there be? The formula to use is *Chang Ning Tang* (Intestine-quieting Decoction):

Radix Angelicae Sinensis (*Dang Gui*), 1 *liang*, washed with wine
Radix Coquitus Rehmanniae (*Shu Di*), 1 *liang*, steamed 9 times
Radix Panacis Ginseng (*Ren Shen*), 3 *qian*
Tuber Ophiopogonis Japonicae (*Mai Dong*), 3 *qian*, cored
Gelatinum Corii Asini (*E Jiao*), 3 *qian*, stir-fried with powdered clam shell
Radix Dioscoreae Oppositae (*Shan Yao*), 3 *qian*, stir-fried
Radix Dipsaci (*Xu Duan*), 2 *qian*
Radix Glycyrrhizae (*Gan Cao*), 1 *qian*
Cortex Cinnamomi (*Rou Gui*), 2 *fen*, sorted & ground

Decoct in water and take. One *ji* (taken), pain is mitigated; a second *ji* (taken), pain is relieved; continuing to take (more *ji*) is more profitable. This is a formula composed of medicinals to supplement the qi and blood, but it supplements qi without risk of over-depressing (the qi), while it supplements blood without the trouble of over-stagnating (the blood). Once qi and blood are generated, without specifically stopping pain, pain is stopped by itself.

Chan Hou Qi Chuan
Postpartum Asthma

Postpartum *chuan,* (asthma, dyspnea, or wheezing) in women is the most critical case of all. Unless treated in a timely fashion, it causes imminent death. About it people only know of qi and blood vacuity, but who would suspect dual desertion of qi and blood? Since both qi and blood desert and the patient is about to die, what on earth can cause the dyspnea? As a matter of fact, it is blood that is on the verge of desertion, while qi has not yet deserted. As the blood is about to desert but the qi is trying to hold it back, (qi) contrarily goes up to cause dyspnea. This is like trying to pick up a drowning person. One's strength may not be equal to the task, but one cannot resign oneself to failure. Therefore, one turns to call upon one's comrades for aid, shouting loudly. This is the *chuan* or dyspnea. Critical as the case may be, it is curable precisely because (the woman) is still capable of dyspnea. The lungs govern the qi. When there is dyspnea, lung qi seems exuberant but is actually debilitated. At this point, blood, which is on the verge of deserting and is, at any rate impossible to generate quickly, is looking very anxiously for the lung qi's coming to its rescue. Whereas the lungs, left with but a tiny amount of qi because of the loss of blood, cannot attend even to themselves. How can they lend a hand to blood? It is a rare case where qi does not desert with the blood. Therefore, in order to rescue the blood, it is necessary to supplement the qi. The formula to use is ***Jiu Tuo Huo Mu Tang*** (Rescue Desertion, Resurrect the Mother Decoction):

Radix Panacis Ginseng (*Ren Shen*), 2 *liang*
Radix Angelicae Sinensis (*Dang Gui*), 1 *liang*, washed with wine
Radix Coquitus Rehmanniae (*Shu Di*), 1 *liang*, steamed 9 times
Fructus Lycii Chinensis (*Gou Qi Zi*), 5 *qian*
Fructus Corni Officinalis (*Shan Yu*), 5 *qian*, steamed, cored

Tuber Ophiopogonis Japonicae (*Ma Dong*), 1 *liang*, cored
Gelatinum Corii Asini (*E Jiao*), 2 *qian*, stir-fried with powdered clam shell
Cortex Cinnamomi (*Rou Gui*), 1 *qian*, sorted & ground
Herba Seu Flos Carbonisatus Schizonepetae Tenuifoliae (*Hei Jie Sui*), 2 *qian*

Decoct in water and take. One *ji* (taken), dyspnea abates; a second *ji* (taken), it mitigates; a third *ji* (taken), it is settled; a fourth *ji* (taken), complete cure is effected. This formula uses Radix Panacis Ginseng to meet and recruit *yuan yang* or original yang. To supplement the qi to the exclusion of the blood, however, will make yang dry and restless. It may succeed in bringing life back for the time being, but this way loss only follows immediately upon gain. On the other hand, supplementing the blood to the exclusion of liver/kidney essence, the root source is not consolidated. In that case, how can yang qi be calmed and increased? Therefore, Radix Coquitus Rehmanniae, Fructus Corni Officinalis, Fructus Lycii Chinensis, and the like are used in addition to greatly supplement the essence of the liver and kidneys and then to greatly boost lung qi. Thus the lung qi becomes sturdy and effulgent and strong enough to up-raise. Due to specific concern that the use of yin-supplementing medicinals postpartum may cause sluggishness and stagnation, Cortex Cinnamomi is added to supplement life-gate fire. This furnishes fire qi with a root and assists Radix Panacis Ginseng in generating qi. In addition, it is able to transport and transform such medicinals as Radix Coquitus Rehmanniae in order to transform essence and generate blood. It is not a safe strategy to assist yang unduly. In that case, blood may, by chance, follow yang and become stirred up and stasis may ascend with it. (Therefore,) Herba Seu Flos Schizonepetae Tenuifoliae is also added to conduct blood back to the channels. Thus lung qi is calmed and dyspnea is soon settled. This treatment is nearly divine.

Chan Hou E Han Shen Chan
Postpartum Aversion to Cold (&) Body Shivering

People suppose that postpartum aversion to cold, trembling or shivering of the body, fever, and thirst in women are the result of postpartum injury (due to) cold. Who would suspect these are due to dual vacuity of the qi and blood and righteous (qi) defeated by evil (qi)? Generally speaking, as long as the qi in the body is not vacuous, it is utterly impossible for evils to invade. (However,) with blood lost in great amounts, the birthing woman must be greatly vacuous of qi. If qi is vacuous, the skin and hair are defenseless and evils naturally find their way quite easily to invade. This does not need an external wind to assail the body. Given any movement, wind may take advantage of vacuity to invade. In terms of a birthing woman, however, it is easy for wind to invade and as easy to leave. (To treat such an) invasion of external evils, generally there is no need to dispel wind. What's more, in birthing women, if there is aversion to cold, this cold is generated in the interior. If there is fever, this heat is due to internal weakness. If there is body trembling or shivering, this trembling is due to qi vacuity. When internal cold is treated, external cold will disperse of itself. When internal weakness is treated, external heat is resolved of itself. When original yang is invigorated, trembling of the body is eliminated of itself. The formula to use is ***Shi Quan Da Bu Tang*** (Ten Complete Great Supplementing Decoction):

Radix Panacis Ginseng (*Ren Shen*), 3 *qian*
Rhizoma Atractylodis Macrocephalae (*Bai Zhu*), 3 *qian*, stir-fried with earth
Sclerotium Poriae Cocoris (*Fu Ling*), 3 *qian*, skinned
Radix Praeparatus Glycyrrhizae (*Zhi Gan Cao*), 1 *qian*

Rhizoma Ligustici Wallichii (*Chuan Xiong*), 1 *qian*, washed with wine
Radix Angelicae Sinensis (*Dang Gui*), 3 *qian*, washed with wine
Radix Coquitus Rehmanniae (*Shu Di*), 5 *qian*, steamed 9 times
Radix Albus Paeoniae Lactiflorae (*Bai Shao*), 2 *qian*, stir-fried with wine
Radix Astragali Seu Hedysari (*Huang Qi*), 1 *liang*, use raw
Cortex Cinnamomi (*Rou Gui*), 1 *qian*, sorted (&) ground

Decoct in water and take. One *ji* will cure all (these) disorders. Because when the righteous is abundant, evils are naturally eliminated, this formula simply supplements vacuity of the qi and blood without dissipating wind or evil repletion. This is all the more so since there is no evil qi (in this case) at all. On account of this, this formula offers a quick cure.

[Several *ji* should be administered in succession. Do not administer only one.]

Chan Hou E Xin Ou Tu
Postpartum Nausea, Retching, (&) Vomiting

Postpartum nausea, the desire to retch, and occasional vomiting in postpartum women is declared by all people to be (due to) cold stomach qi. Who would suspect cold kidney qi? The stomach serves as the pass to the kidney. When cold, stomach qi is unable to move to the kidneys; while kidney qi, when cold, is unable to move to the stomach. Because of this, the kidneys and stomach are inseparable. In terms of the puerperium, however, excessive loss of blood is bound to lead to dried up kidney water. When kidney water is dried up, kidney fire flames upward and the stomach should not be troubled by cold. Then why do the kidneys become cold and why also does the stomach become cold? If, shortly after delivery, water just dries up abruptly, vacuity fire is not yet generated.

Because fire is not yet generated, cold phenomena naturally show themselves. The appropriate treatment method is to supplement the fire in the kidneys. If, however, this is not assisted by water, fire would be over water, and, most likely, there would arise the pattern of stirring fire with yin vacuity. (Therefore,) it is necessary to incorporate fire-supplementation into water(-supplementation) and to incorporate stomach-warming into kidney(-warming). Then the kidneys will be rid of the trouble of excessive heat, while the stomach has the pleasure of being assisted. The formula to use is ***Wen Wei Zhi Ou Tang*** (Warm the Kidneys, Stop Retching Decoction):

Radix Coquitus Rehmanniae (*Shu Di*), 5 *qian*, steamed 9 times
Radix Morindae Officinalis (*Ba Ji*), 1 *liang*, soaked in salt water
Radix Panacis Ginseng (*Ren Shen*), 3 *qian*
Rhizoma Atractylodis Macrocephalae (*Bai Zhu*), 1 *liang*, stir-fried with earth
Fructus Corni Officinalis (*Shan Yu*), 5 *qian*, steamed, cored
Rhizoma Praeparata Zingiberis (*Pao Jiang*), 1 *qian*
Sclerotium Poriae Cocoris (*Fu Ling*), 2 *qian*, skinned
Exocarpium Citri Rubri (*Ju Hong*), 5 *fen*, washed with ginger juice
Fructus Amomi Cardamomi (*Bai Kou*), 1 piece, ground

Decoct in water and take. One *ji* (taken), retching and vomiting are stopped; a second *ji* (taken), they will never recur; a fourth *ji* (taken), and complete cure is effected. In this formula, there are more kidney-supplementing medicinals than stomach-treating ingredients. However, treating the kidneys is as good as treating the stomach. Therefore, when the kidney qi soars, stomach cold is resolved naturally. There is no need to employ greatly hot medicinals to warm the stomach to dispel cold.

[This formula should not be administered till the lochia has run out completely. Nau$ea with desire to retch arising one or two days after parturition is due to up-surging of the lochia. It is proper, (therefore,) to administer *Jia Wei Sheng Hua Tang* (Added Flavors Generating & Transforming Decoction): Radix Angelicae Sinensis (*Quan Dang Gui*), 1 *liang*, washed with wine; Rhizoma Ligustici Wallichii (*Chuan Xiong*), 2 *qian*; Rhizoma Praeparata Zingiberis (*Pao Jiang*), 1 *qian*; Fructus Carbonisatus Crataegi (*Dong Zha Tan*), 2 *qian*; Semen Pruni Persicae (*Tao Ren*), 1 *qian*, ground; to be decocted with 1 cup of Shaoxing wine mixed with 3 cups of water.]

Chan Hou Xue Beng
Postpartum Profuse (Uterine) Bleeding

Xue beng or profuse (uterine) bleeding with clouding and dizziness in young women arising half a month after delivery is declared by all people to be (due to) malign blood surging into the heart. Who would suspect that it is caused by indiscreet sexual intercouse? Although (the situation) over half a month (after delivery) is different from that two or three days after parturition, qi and blood, which are just beginning to generate, are not yet completely recovered. Even though the blood passageways are clean, the *bao tai* has not yet recovered from damage and injury and, therefore, it is absolutely imperative not to try (sexual intercourse) which might cause new damage to the gates. *Xue beng* with clouding and dizziness resulting from negligence of abstention and (self-)nursing at the preliminary stage of recovery of qi and blood is (ascribed) not only to damaged gate of the *bao tai* but also dual injury of the heart and kidneys. When essence is drained and spirit has deserted, there is no other good choice but to greatly supplement the qi and blood. The formula to use is ***Jiu Bai Qiu Sheng Tang*** (Rescue Collapse, Rekindle Life Decoction):

Radix Panacis Ginseng (*Ren Shen*), 2 *liang*
Radix Angelicae Sinensis (*Dang Gui*), 2 *liang*, washed with wine
Rhizoma Atractylodis Macrocephalae (*Bai Zhu*), 2 *liang*, stir-fried with earth
Radix Coquitus Rehmanniae (*Shu Di*), 1 *liang*, steamed 9 times
Fructus Corni Officinalis (*Shan Yu*), 5 *qian*, steamed
Radix Dioscoreae Oppositae (*Shan Yao*), 5 *qian*, stir-fried
Semen Zizyphi Spinosae (*Zao Ren*), 5 *qian*, use raw
Radix Praeparatus Aconiti Carmichaeli (*Fu Zi*), 1 *fen* or 1 *qian*, self-prepared

Decoct in water and take. One *ji* (taken, and) the spirit is stabilized; a second *ji* (taken), dizziness is stopped; a third *ji* (taken), bleeding is stopped. If the first *ji* takes effect, administer three or four more *ji* in succession. At this point, reduce the dosage by half and administer ten more *ji*. Then resurrection can be celebrated. This formula supplements the qi to recover original yang from the home of nothingness. Once yang is recovered, qi is recovered and is naturally (able) to contain the blood, welcome back the spirit, and generate essence to resume life.

[There are also cases where the central qi has become vacuous with incessant, profuse (uterine) bleeding occurring immediately after delivery and with it qi deserts. This is an extremely critical case. Failure to save life counts eight or nine out of ten cases. The one or two cases (which are saved) are saved entirely by *Du Shen Tang* (Solitary Ginseng Decoction, composed of) 5 *qian* of Radix Panacis Ginseng (*Ren Shen*), stemmed, smashed, (and) decocted rapidly. If there is any delay, the qi will desert. (Therefore,) there is no time to lose. After the decoction has been prepared, pour it slowly (down the throat of the patient), and, when qi is back, decoct and administer another *ji*. For other treatment methods, refer to the chapter entitled *xue beng*. However, in postpartum cases, Radix Albus

Carbonisatus Paeoniae Lactiflorae (*Hang Shao Tan*) and various (other) cooling medicinals should not be used. Such cases are all caused by sexual intercourse one or two days before delivery. Refrain from this!]

Chan Hou Shou Shang Bao Tai Lin Li Bu Zhi Postpartum Incessant Dribbling (of Blood Due to) the *Bao Tai* Being Injured by Hand

In the course of giving birth, some women's *bao tai* is injured by the midwife who has put her hand into the birth gate. As a result, (blood) dribbles incessantly and cannot be stopped for a moment. People assert that a broken uterus is not mendable, but, in fact, it is. Since injured skin can be mended, why should injuries inside the abdomen alone not be treatable? Some may argue that injuries in the exterior may be cured by external treatment with medicinals to generate the skin. While, for wounds in the interior, there is no way to apply salvaging or mending even though there exists a cure-all medicinal paste. For wounds in the interior, it is true that external treatments are not possible, but does internal treatment necessarily fail to achieve effect (in such cases)? Think of the toxins of ulcerous wounds. Since even they can (be helped to) grow flesh by means of administering medication, what kind of difficulty is there in healing this damage or defect which is but a slight detriment without any malign toxin and is caused merely by carelessness during parturition? The formula to use is ***Wan Bao Yin*** (Renew the Uterus Drink):

Radix Panacis Ginseng (*Ren Shen*), 1 *liang*
Rhizoma Atractylodis Macrocephalae (*Bai Zhu*), 10 *liang*, stir-fried with earth
Sclerotium Poriae Cocoris (*Fu Ling*), 3 *qian*, skinned
Radix Astragali Seu Hedysari (*Sheng Huang Qi*), 5 *qian*

Radix Angelicae Sinensis (*Dang Gui*), 1 *liang*, stir-fried with wine
Rhizoma Ligustici Wallichii (*Chuan Xiong*), 5 *qian*
Pulvis Rhizomatis Bletillae Striatae (*Bai Ji Mo*), 1 *qian*
Flos Carthami Tinctorii (*Hong Hua*), 1 *qian*
Herba Leonuri Heterophylli (*Yi Mu Cao*), 3 *qian*
Semen Pruni Persicae (*Tao Ren*), 10 pieces, soaked, stir-fried, (&) ground

Boil a pig's or sheep's urinary bladder and then decoct the drugs (in the soup). Ten *ji* taken on an empty stomach, (and) complete cure is effected. In case of injured uterus, it is appropriate to use uterus-supplementing medicinals, so why are qi and blood supplementing medicinals used here instead? In the course of delivery, it is naturally not permissible to probe with the hands. But, (in this case,) the midwife has and so has injured the uterus. This must have been because of difficult delivery, and a difficult delivery is due to qi and blood vacuity. Serious postpartum injury of the qi and blood adds to this vacuity. Vacuity was the cause of injury and this injury, in turn, has worsened this vacuity. Apart from greatly supplementing qi and blood, what else is effective for a broken uterus? Greatly supplementing qi and blood is just like offering food to the hungry or drink to the thirsty. Thus the *jing shen* or essence spirit will be greatly enhanced; while qi and blood will be produced again. Therefore, what kind of difficulty is there in renewing the uterus? Hence success is achieved in no more than ten days.

Can Hou Si Zhi Fu Zhong Postpartum Swelling (&) Edema of the Four Limbs

Postpartum swelling and edema of the four limbs, alternating cold and heat, dyspnea, coughing, inhibited chest and diaphragm, acid regurgitation, and lateral costal pain are declared by all people to be (due to) vanquished blood running into the channels and connecting vessels and percolating into the limbs. This, (then,) results in qi counterflow. Who would suspect dual vacuity of the liver and kidneys and failure of yin to leave yang? In the postpartum woman, qi and blood are seriously depleted and it is natural that kidney water is insufficient and that kidney fire is boisterous. Water, when insufficient, is unable to nurture the liver. When liver/wood becomes excessively dry and wood is lacking in fluids, dry wood catches fire. (In this case,) kidney fire finds an associate, and both the mother and child burn. Flames surge straight up to restrain lung/metal above. Being tormented by fire, metal has no strength left to overwhelm the liver. In consequence, the problems of coughing, dyspnea, and fullness arise. If liver fire becomes effulgent and goes down to restrain spleen/earth, earth, tormented by wood, has no strength left to overwhelm water. In consequence, the problem of swollen limbs appears. However, this effulgent fire of liver/wood is only a false appearance. This fire is not really effulgent. Falsely effulgent qi seems exuberant, but, in fact, it is insufficient. Therefore, sometimes there occurs fever and sometimes cold. These come and go in an unpredictable way depending on the waxing and waning of qi. This cold is not true cold, (and) this heat is not true heat. They are (manifestations of) unsoothed qi due to counterflow between the chest and the diaphragm. The lateral costal regions are where the liver is located and acidity is the qi flavor of the liver. Acid regurgitation and lateral costal pain are both manifestations of liver vacuity and the kidneys' lack of ability to flourish. The appropriate treatment method is to supplement the blood to nurture the liver and supplement the essence to generate the blood. When essence and blood are made abundant, qi becomes normal by itself and all problems, such as cold and heat, coughing and water swelling will disappear. The formula to use is ***Zhuan Qi Tang*** (Rectify the Qi Decoction):

Radix Panacis Ginseng (*Ren Shen*), 3 *qian*
Sclerotium Poriae Cocoris (*Fu Ling*), 3 *qian*, skinned
Rhizoma Atractylodis Macrocephalae (*Bai Zhu*), 3 *qian*, stir-fried with earth
Radix Angelicae Sinensis (*Dang Gui*), 5 *qian*, washed with wine
Radix Albus Paeoniae Lactiflorae (*Bai Shao*), 5 *qian*, stir-fried with wine
Radix Coquitus Rehmanniae (*Shu Di*), 1 *liang*, steamed 9 times
Fructus Corni Officinalis (*Shan Yu*), 3 *qian*, steamed
Radix Dioscoreae Oppositae (*Shan Yao*), 5 *qian*, stir-fried
Semen Euryalis Ferocis (*Qian Shi*), 3 *qian*, stir-fried
Radix Bupleuri (*Chai Hu*), 5 *fen*
Fructus Psoraleae Corylifoliae (*Gu Zhi*), 1 *qian*, stir-fried with salt water

Decoct in water and take. Three *ji* (and there is some) effect, (while) 10 *ji* effect a cure. This formula is composed entirely of blood-supplementing, essence-supplementing ingredients. Then why is it named qi-rectifying? It should be understood that qi counterflow results from qi vacuity or, rather, vacuity of liver and kidney qi. Supplementing the essence and blood of the liver and kidneys is as good as supplementing the qi of the liver and kidneys. Vacuity leads to counterflow, while effulgence leads to normalization. Therefore, supplementation is rectifying. Once qi is rectified, all the disorders will cure and, once yin leaves yang, the trouble of interference between yin and yang will disappear.

[This formula is so perfect that it allows for no modification. It is proper to use slightly charred Radix Albus Paeoniae Lactiflorae.]

Chan Hou Rou Xian Chu
Postpartum Exit of Fleshy Fiber

(Some) women after delivery have a fleshy fiber or thread 2-3 *chi* (or feet) long exit from the water passageway. This fiber or thread gives a deadly pain when touched. People suppose this to be the prolapsed *bao tai* or uterus. Who would suspect vacuity desertion of the *dai mai*? The *dai mai* binds the conception and the governing vessels, the former in front and the latter in back. When these two vessels are strong, the *dai mai* is solid and firm. When they are flaccid, the *dai mai* collapses and sags. Owing to excessive postpartum loss of blood, there is no blood to nurture the conception or governing vessels. As the *dai mai* collapses and sags, left with no strength to raise itself up, it follows the urine out. Sagging of the *dai mai* usually gives pain in the lumbar and umbilical regions. What's worse, the *dai mai* has prolapsed beyond the birth gate, way too far out of position. How can it not cause a deadly pain? The formula to use is ***Liang Shou Tang*** (Dual Withdrawing Decoction):

Radix Panacis Ginseng (*Ren Shen*), 1 *liang*
Rhizoma Atractylodis Macrocephalae (*Bai Zhu*), 2 *liang*, stir-fried with earth
Rhizoma Ligustici Wallichii (*Chuan Xiong*), 3 *qian*, washed with wine
Radix Coquitus Rehmanniae steamed 9 times (*Jiu Zheng Shu Di*), 2 *liang*

Radix Dioscoreae Oppositae (*Shan Yao*), 1 *liang*, stir-fried
Fructus Corni Officinalis (*Shan Yu*), 4 *qian*, steamed
Semen Euryalis Ferocis (*Qian Shi*), 5 *qian*, stir-fried
Semen Dolichoris Lablabis (*Bian Dou*), 5 *qian*, stir-fried
Radix Morindae Officinalis (*Ba Ji*), 3 *qian*, soaked in salt water
Cortex Eucommiae Ulmoidis (*Du Zhong*), 5 *qian*, char-fried
Semen Ginkgonis Bilobae (*Bai Guo*), 10 pieces, pounded

Decoct in water. One *ji* (and) withdrawal is half accomplished; 2 *ji* (and) withdrawal is complete. The reason that this formula (is designed to) supplement not only the conception and governing vessels but also the lumbus and umbilicus is that these two vessels are linked with them. If the *ren* and *du* were supplemented to the exclusion of the lumbus and umbilicus, these two vessels would have no backing. Then how could the *dai mai* be up-lifted? Only if dual supplementation is applied can the *ren* and *du* procure aid from the lumbus and umbilicus so the *dai mai* can withdraw by the strength of these two vessels.

[This formula is able to treat kidney vacuity, lumbago, and enuresis. It should not be underestimated.]

Chan Hou Gan Wei
Postpartum Liver Atony

From the orifice of the vagina in (some) postpartum women may be suspended a thing, handkerchief-shaped, possibly with corners or two branches. People suppose this to be (due to) parturient breakdown. Who would suspect that it is due to *gan wei* or liver atony? And how does this liver atony develop after delivery? Because of injury resulting from overtaxation and overwork before delivery and, in addition, an outburst of savage anger, the liver is unable to store blood and blood is lost excessively. As a result, the fatty membrane of the liver collapses and prolapses accompanied by bleeding. In shape, it is like but it is not the uterus. If it were the uterus that prolapsed, it would show an eggplant shape and reach but never outreach the birth gate. It is only the fatty membrane of the liver that can typically come out of the birth gate. This can be as long as 6 or 7 *cun* outside and sometimes stick to the mat, dried, covering a spot the size the palm. If it were the prolapsed uterus, the patient would have suffered instant death. How could she come to life again? The appropriate treatment method is to greatly supplement the qi and blood in addition to a small amount of up-raising ingredients. Thus, liver qi is made effulgent and becomes easy to generate; while liver blood is made effulgent and becomes easy to nurture. When the liver gains strength by virtue of this generation and nurturing, this fatty membrane will withdraw of itself. The formula to use is ***Shou Mo Tang*** (Withdraw the Membrane Decoction):

Radix Astragali Seu Hedysari (*Sheng Huang Qi*), 1 *liang*
Radix Panacis Ginseng (*Ren Shen*), 5 *qian*
Rhizoma Atractylodis Macrocephalae (*Bai Zhu*), 5 *qian*, stir-fried with earth
Radix Angelicae Sinensis (*Dang Gui*), 3 *qian*, washed with wine
Rhizoma Cimicifugae (*Sheng Ma*), 1 *qian*
Radix Albus Paeoniae Lactiflorae (*Bai Shao*), 5 *qian*, scorch-fried with wine

Decoct in water and take. One *ji* will withdraw (the membrane). It may be asked why this formula proves (so) effective in spite of making use of Radix Albus Paeoniae Lactiflorae, since its use is contraindicated postpartum for fear that it might quell the source of qi generation? (Whoever raises this question) must not have read (Zhang) Zhong-jing's works. Oho! The reason that Radix Albus Paeoniae Lactiflorae is not allowed to be used frequently in postpartum cases is fear that it will promote contraction of stasis. But it is wrong to assert that it quells the source of qi generation. It should not be (universally) excluded, particularly when the problem is in the liver. Furthermore, when used together with large amounts of qi and blood supplementing (ingredients), it forgets its sour contraction. What trouble can it make then? And, in the case of prolapsed fatty membrane, it is just by the strength of its sour contraction that it helps Rhizoma Cimicifugae to raise the qi and blood and that (such) a rapid effect is achieved.

[The withdrawal of the liver membrane is entirely due to Radix Albus Paeoniae Lactiflorae. It should not be administered charred.]

Chan Hou Qi Xue Liang Xu Ru Ye Bu Xia Postpartum Qi (&) Blood Dual Vacuity Breast Milk Not Descending

After delivery, (some) women do not have a drop of breast milk. People suppose (this to be due to) blocked milk ducts. Who would suspect dual drying up of qi and blood? Milk is a product of the transformation of qi and blood. Certainly milk cannot be produced without blood, but it also cannot be without qi. In comparison, blood transforms milk less speedily than qi does. In the newly birthed woman, blood is too depleted to look after itself. (Therefore,) how can it transform milk? It is entirely due to the strength of the qi that blood is moved to transform milk. That the breasts have secreted not a drop of milk for several days since delivery clearly reveals a shortage of blood and debility of qi. When qi is effulgent, milk is effulgent. When qi is debilitated, milk is debilitated. When qi is dried up, milk is dried up. It must be of necessity so. Ignorant of the importance of greatly supplementing qi and blood, people nowadays know no better than to promote lactation. It should be understood that without qi, milk has nothing to transform it and, without blood, milk has nothing from which to be produced. The appropriate treatment method is to supplement qi to generate blood. Thus, breast milk will flow by itself and there is no need to disinhibit the portals to promote lactation. The formula is called ***Tong Ru Dan*** (Open the Breasts Elixir):

Radix Panacis Ginseng (*Ren Shen*), 1 *liang*
Radix Astragali Seu Hedysari (*Sheng Huang Qi*), 1 *liang*
Radix Angelicae Sinensis (*Dang Gui*), 2 *liang*, washed with wine
Tuber Ophiopogonis Japonicae (*Mai Dong*), 5 *qian*, cored
Caulis Akebiae Mutong (*Mu Tong*), 3 *fen*
Radix Platycodis Grandiflori (*Jie Geng*), 3 *fen*
Ham hock (*Qi Kong Zhu Ti*), 2 hocks, unshod

Decoct in water and take. Two *ji* will have milk gushing like a spring. This formula exclusively supplements the qi and blood to produce breast milk. This is because there are no other producers of the milk than the qi and blood. There is no comparison between the absence of breast milk due to postpartum drying up of qi and blood and that due to blocked milk ducts. This formula, though not (composed of medicinals) to promote lactation, is called a breast-opening elixir because administering it is capable of promoting lactation. Because it does not open the breasts but generates milk, it is also alright to call it *Sheng Ru Dan* (Milk Generating Elixir).

Chan Hou Yu Jie Ru Ye Bu Tong
Postpartum Depression (&) Knotting Breast Milk Not Flowing Freely

After delivery, (some) strong young women, who may have overheard some unpleasant remarks, experience breast distention, fullness, and pain with stoppage of the breast milk's flow. People suppose (this to be due to) fire heat of the *yang ming*. Who would suspect liver qi depression and binding or knotting? The *yang ming* is ascribed to the stomach, a bowel abundant in both qi and blood. Transformation of breast milk is the responsibility of the *yang ming* which belongs to earth. In strong women, though blood has collapsed after delivery, the qi of the *yang ming* is, practically (speaking), not utterly debilitated. However, it cannot transform milk unless its flow is freed by the qi of liver/wood. Therefore, the *yang ming* is but partly at fault. Transformation of milk does not depend on the blood but entirely upon the qi. If several days have passed since delivery, there should be milk. Distention, fullness, and pain in the breasts show a tendency but failure to transform milk. What else could cause this if not depressed qi? (In such cases,) it is apparent that there exists depression induced by shame and indignation and that earth and wood are bound by each other. How then can milk be transformed to produce a flow? The appropriate treatment method is to greatly soothe liver/wood qi. Thus the qi and blood of the *yang ming* are naturally freed and the flow of milk will, consequently, also be freed. (Therefore,) there is no need to specially free it. The formula is called ***Tong Gan Sheng Ru Tang*** (Free the Liver, Generate Milk Decoction):

Radix Albus Paeoniae Lactiflorae (*Bai Shao*), 5 *qian*, stir-fried with vinegar
Radix Angelicae Sinensis (*Dang Gui*), 5 *qian*, washed with wine
Rhizoma Atractylodis Macrocephalae (*Bai Zhu*), 5 *qian*, stir-fried with earth
Radix Coquitus Rehmanniae (*Shu Di*), 3 *fen*
Radix Glycyrrhizae (*Gan Cao*), 3 *fen*
Tuber Ophiopogonis Japonicae (*Mai Dong*), 5 *qian*, cored
Medulla Tetrapanacis Papyriferi (*Tong Cao*), 1 *qian*
Radix Bupleuri (*Chai Hu*), 1 *qian*

Radix Polygalae Tenuifoliae (*Yuan Zhi*), 1 *qian*

Decoct in water and take. One *ji* will free the flow; a second *ji* is needless.

[When stir-fried with millet, Tuber Ophiopogonis Japonicae, far from cooling the stomach, will be directly led into it by the flavor of the grain and (thus) transform milk more rapidly.]

Book 3

Chan Hou
Birthing & Afterwards

Chapter 1

Chan Hou Zong Lun An Overview of Postpartum (Disorders)

Diseases that are occasioned by qi and blood debility and by spleen and stomach vacuity (tend to) deteriorate after delivery. For that reason, in dealing with postpartum disorders, Mr. Dan-xi advocated giving priority to greatly supplementing the qi and blood and treating other problems only subsidiarily.[1] This statement by him embraces (all) the principles of handling postpartum disorders. Applying it to the design of formulas, (one) will be free from errors in handling parturient cases.

Postpartum worry, fright, taxation, fatigue, and sudden vacuity of qi and blood provide a chance for various conditions to take advantage of vacuity and easily enter. If there is qi (*i.e.*, qi depression), do not apply only consuming-dissipation. If there is food (*i.e.*, food injury or food accumulation), do not apply only abducting-dispersion. In case of heat, do not use Radix Scutellariae Baicalensis (*Huang Qin*) or Rhizoma Coptidis Chinensis (*Huang Lian*). In case of cold, do not use Cortex Cinnamomi (*Rou Gui*) or Radix Praeparatus Aconiti Carmichaeli

---

1 Dan-Xi Xian Sheng, Mr. or Prof. Dan-xi, refers to Zhu Zhen-heng, styled Dan-xi, one of the so-called Four Great Masters of the Jin-Yuan. Zhu Dan-xi was the founder of the School of Enriching Yin which emphasized supplementation of yin to control hyperactivity of yang.

(*Fu Zi*). Cold leads to blood clots, stoppage, and stagnation. Heat leads to new blood flooding and flowing. As to central vacuity with external invasion, abundant (evidence of) exterior patterns of the three yang seems to warrant diaphoresis, but, in postpartum cases, use of *Ma Huang (Tang,* Ephedra Decoction, only) inflicts double exhaustion of yang. Abundant (evidence of) interior patterns of the three yin seems to warrant precipitation or purgation, but, in postpartum cases, use of *Cheng Qi (Tang,* Qi-supporting Decoction, only) causes double collapse of yin (and) blood. In cases of deafness and lateral costal pain which are (caused by) retention of lochia due to kidney vacuity, do not use *Chai Hu (Tang,* Bupleurum Decoction). Delirious speech with perspiration, a condition of origin weakness (*yuan ruo*) similar to that of evils (*i.e.*, replete evils) should not be (treated) as stomach repletion. In case of inversion which is due to debilitated yang, be it cold or hot, to recover yang and convalesce from weakness, there is no other choice but to apply great supplementation. In case of tetany which is due to depletion of yin/blood, be it hard or soft, to soothe the sinews and activate the connecting vessels, there is no other choice but to enrich the *ying*. Alternating fever and chills with attacks at irregular intervals are similar to the manifestations of malaria, but, if they are treated as malaria, they will hang on and become difficult to cure. Nonsensical speech with spirit failing to keep to its abode looks like a condition of evils (*i.e.*, replete evils). If it is treated as (replete) evils, crisis and death are to be expected.

Dry, bound stools due to excessive loss of blood can be treated by adding Herba Cistanchis (*Rou Cong Rong*) to *Sheng Hua Tang* (Generating & Transforming Decoction) to free it. They are beyond the intestine-moistening *Cheng Qi (Tang)*. In case of short, inhibited voidings of urine due to excessive sweating,

Liu Jun Zi Tang (Six Gentlemen Decoction)[2] with a double amount of Radix Panacis Ginseng (*Ren Shen*) and Radix Astragali Seu Hedysari (*Huang Qi*) is capable of generating fluids and assisting humor to effect disinhibition. *Jia Shen Sheng Hua Tang* (Generating & Transforming Decoction with added Ginseng), taken at short intervals, can rescue postpartum crises. *Chang Sheng Huo Ming Dan* (Long Life, Life-Saving Elixir)[3], taken frequently, can resurrect a patient who has been fasting. *Tui shan*[4] and prolapse of the rectum, which are usually due to qi vacuity and falling, are (indications of) *Bu Zhong Yi Qi Tang* (Supplement the Center, Boost the Qi Decoction). Clenched jaws and hypertonicity of the fists, which are caused by dry blood and quasi-wind(stroke), are (indications of) *Jia Shen Sheng Hua Tang* (Generating & Transforming Decoction with added Ginseng). For serious pain in the birth gate due to the inroads of wind, it is proper to administer the *Qiang Huo Yang Rong Tang* (Notopterygium Nurture Construction Decoction).[5] Cool injury (*shang liang*) of the jade gate[6] and failure to shut or close is best treated by washing with *Ma Er Huang Liu San.*[7] (To treat) racing of the heart and fright palpitations, *Sheng Hua Tang* can stabilize orientation. (To

---

2 The ingredients of this formula include Radix Panacis Ginseng (*Ren Shen*), Rhizoma Atractylodis Macrocephalae (*Bai Zhu*), Sclerotium Poriae Cocoris (*Fu Ling*), Radix Glycyrrhizae (*Gan Cao*), Rhizoma Pinelliae Ternatae (*Ban Xia*), and Pericarpium Citri Reticulatae (*Chen Pi*).

3 Ingredients unknown

4 A sagging sensation and pain in the sides of the lower abdomen.

5 Ingredients unknown

6 A poetic name for the vaginal orifice

7 Identification unknown. Two of the ingredients seem to be Acacia Catechu (*Er Cha*) and Sulphur (*Liu Huang*).

treat) abstraction as if spell-bound, *An Shen Wan* (Calm the Spirit Pill)[8] should be helped by *Gui Pi (Tang).*[9] In case of oppression, fullness, and empty vexation due to qi (depression), Radix Saussureae Seu Vladimiriae (*Mu Xiang*) can be added as an assistant to *Sheng Hua Tang.* (To treat) acid belching and aversion to food due to food (accumulation), it is better to add Massa Medica Fermentata (*Shen Qu*) and Fructus Germinatus Hordei Vulgaris (*Mai Ya*) to *Liu Jun Zi (Tang).*

Lignum Sappanis (*Su Mu*) and Rhizoma Curcumae Zedoariae (*E Zhu*) are particularly capable of breaking blood. Pericarpium Viridis Citri Reticulatae (*Qing Pi*) and Fructus Citri Seu Ponciri (*Zhi Qiao*) are most capable of dispersing fullness and distention. All qi-consuming and blood-cracking medicinals and diaphoresis, ejection, diffusion, and precipitation methods are (usually) applied in the strong and repletion cases but not in case of pregnancy or postpartum. In terms of a case shortly after delivery, as a rule, it is necessary above all (else) to enquire about the lochia. If there is lump pain not yet relieved, do not use Radix Panacis Ginseng and Rhizoma Atractylodis Macrocephalae hastily. (However,) after relief of abdominal pain, supplementing the center and boosting the qi are past questioning about (*i.e.*, they are axiomatic). As to desertion sweating due to yang collapse and distressed rapid dyspneic

---

8 This formula is composed of Rhizoma Coptidis Chinensis (*Huang Lian*), 2 *qian;* Cinnabaris (*Zhu Sha*), 1 *qian;* Radix Rehmanniae (*Sheng Di*), 1.5 *qian;* Radix Angelicae Sinensis (*Dang Gui*), 1.5 *qian;* and Radix Glycyrrhizae (*Gan Cao*), 1.5 *qian.*

9 The ingredients of this formula include Radix Panacis Ginseng (*Ren Shen*), Radix Astragali Seu Hedysari (*Huang Qi*), Radix Angelicae Sinensis (*Dang Gui*), Arillus Euphoriae Longanae (*Long Yan Rou*), Rhizoma Atractylodis Macrocephalae (*Bai Zhu*), Radix Saussureae Seu Vladimiriae (*Mu Xiang*), Sclerotium Poriae Cocoris (*Fu Ling*), Radix Polygalae Tenuifoliae (*Yuan Zhi*), Semen Zizyphi Spinosae (*Suan Zao Ren*), Radix Praeparatus Glycyrrhizae (*Zhi Gan Cao*), Rhizoma Recens Zingiberis (*Sheng Jiang*), and Fructus Zizyphi Jujubae (*Da Zao*).

breathing, take frequently *Jia Shen Sheng Hua Tang*. It serves as an expedient measure. But, where yin collapse with fire/heat and profuse (uterine) bleeding with inversion and dizziness are concerned, boil without delay the original *Sheng Hua Tang* for emergency treatment.

Wang Tai-pu[10] said,

> To treat the lower, supplement the lower with (the right choice between) slow and swift treatment (methods). The slow clears the roads but is small in strength, while the swift is thick in flavor and massive in strength.

To treat postpartum disorders, it is proper to follow (Zhu) Dan-xi to secure the root. As to the method of administration, it is proper to follow Tai-pu in administering at short intervals.

Entrusted with a matter of life and death, one should always focus on (and anticipate) the most critical condition. If one is to be free from any fault in treating, one must concentrate on what is obscure. This work does not exhaust postpartum conditions, but it will hopefully be of some value since each case study is supported by the evidence of clinical experience (gathered) in the countryside.

---

10 Wang is the family name; Tai-pu was the title of an office in charge of the royal chariots, stables, and pastures. This refers to Wang Bing (710-804 CE), a senior minister at the court, who took 12 years to edit and compile the *Huang Di Nei Jing (Yellow Emperor's Internal Classic)*.

Chapter 2

Chan Qian Hou Fang Zheng Yi Ji Indications (&) Contraindications of Pre (&) Postpartum Disorders

Zheng Chan Normal Delivery

(In) normal delivery, intermittent abdominal pain with lumbar and lateral costal aching pain or urgency with the placenta still intact is called *nong tai* or playing fetus. Administration of *Ba Zhen Tang Jia Xiang Fu* (Eight Pearls Decoction with added Cyperus)[1] will surely calm. In case of mild pain lingering several days after the breaking of the placenta, administer the above medicinals and wait.

Shang Chan Injured Delivery

(In) *shang chan* or injured delivery, injury or stirring of the *tai* or fetus before sufficient moons (*i.e.*, before full term), abdomi-

---

1 The ingredients in this formula include Radix Panacis Ginseng (*Ren Shen*), Sclerotium Poriae Cocoris (*Fu Ling*), Rhizoma Atractylodis Macrocephalae (*Bai Zhu*), Radix Glycyrrhizae (*Gan Cao*), Rhizoma Ligustici Wallichii (*Chuan Xiong*), Radix Angelicae Sinensis (*Dang Gui*), Radix Albus Paeoniae Lactiflorae (*Bai Shao*), Radix Coquitus Rehmanniae (*Di Huang*).

nal and periumbilical pain, too early administration of birth-hastening medicinals, or overexertion of the mother may (all) force the child to deviate from position so as to render natural delivery impossible. Therefore, towards childbirth, the mother should behave in a leisurely way and try to refrain from oversleep, overeating, and wine. When she feels (the fetus) turning in the womb, she should lie on her back to wait for the fetus to turn in position. It is better to be cautious in advance than to have trouble in the end.

Tiao Chan
Balancing (or Regulating) Delivery

(In terms of) balancing or regulating delivery, towards childbirth, select the midwife, ready the (necessary) instruments and utensils, and procure medicinals like Radix Panacis Ginseng (*Ren Shen*) to have in store. During delivery, the presence of many people making noise is not allowed. (The birthing woman) can be supported by two persons or she may be allowed to stand alone (supporting herself) against something. In case of heart vexation, take a spoonful of honey dissolved in boiling water, but it is better to administer *Du Huo Tang* (Angelica Duhuo & Notopterygium Decoction).[2] When hungry, take a little porridge. (The woman) should not let (herself) go hungry or thirsty. In case of difficult delivery, just

---

2 The ingredients in this formula consist of Radix Notopterygii (*Qiang Huo*), Radix Angelicae Duhuo (*Du Huo*), Radix Ledebouriellae Sesloidis (*Fang Feng*), Rhizoma Ligustici Wallichii (*Chuan Xiong*), Radix Angelicae Sinensis (*Dang Gui*), Herba Cum Radice Asari Sieboldi (*Xi Xin*), Cortex Cinnamomi (*Rou Gui*), Radix Panacis Ginseng (*Ren Shen*), Rhizoma Pinelliae Ternatae (*Ban Xia*), Rhizoma Acori Graminei (*Shi Chang Pu*), Sclerotium Pararadicis Poriae Cocoris (*Fu Shen*), Radix Polygalae Tenuifoliae (*Yuan Zhi*), Radix Cynanchi Atrati (*Bai Wei*), 5 *qian* each, and Radix Praeparatus Glycyrrhizae (*Zhi Gan Cao*), 2.5 *qian*. Grind these and mix together. Take with Rhizoma Zingiberis (*Sheng Jiang*) and Fructus Zizyphi Jujubae (*Da Zao*). Dose: 1 *liang*.

pretend and say that it is due to birthing twins or non-descension of the placenta. The birthing mother should be kept free from fright or scare.

Cui Sheng
Hastening Birth

(In terms of) *cui sheng* or hastening birth, in case of fatigue and sleepiness with difficult delivery due to sitting on the straw earlier than necessary, administer *Ba Zhen Tang* with a small amount of Rhizoma Cyperi Rotundi (*Xiang Fu*) and Gummum Olibani (*Ru Xiang*) to assist the blood and qi. *Ba Zhen Tang* can also be used in case of an early broken placenta with humor and blood already dried.

Dong Chan
Frozen Delivery

Dong chan or frozen delivery (is due to) heavenly cold (*i.e.*, cold weather causing) the blood and qi to be congealed and stagnant, thus birthing is not able to be rapid. Therefore, (the birthing woman) should be warmly clothed and placed in a warm chamber. The heart and upper back as well as the lower body should be kept particularly warm.

Re Chan
Hot Delivery

(In terms of) *re chan* or hot delivery, in hot months, warmth and coolness should be suitably adjusted. If the chamber is crowded, hot oppressing steam may cause headache with a red facial complexion, clouding and dizziness, and so forth. It is appropriate to drink a little cool water to resolve (these disorders). It is, however, necessary to keep off wind, rain, or clammy coolness.

Heng Chan
Transverse Delivery

(In terms of) *heng chan* or transverse delivery, the baby lies in the mother's abdomen with head up and feet down. In the process of delivery, it turns head downward. If the birthing mother exerts herself to force it, the child will stop turning half way in a crosswise or transverse position. The mother should be told to lie calmly on her back to allow the child to turn to the right position by itself. If the fetus becomes entangled in the umbilical cord, the midwife may take hold of the fetus by the shoulder with her middle finger. (In this case,) use birth-hastening medicinals and push with strength (and the child) will be delivered.

(Take) Radix Angelicae Sinensis (*Dang Gui*) and Fructus Perillae Frutescentis (*Zi Su*), 3 *qian* each, boiled in river water (and the child will) presently come down.

Another method (is to) rub (with water) a good quality ink stick (on an ink stone) and drink (the ink). (The child will) presently come down.

(Yet) another method (is to) take Herba Leonuri Heterophylli (*Yi Mu Cao*), 6 *liang*, boiled down thick in water and mixed with a big cup of a child's urine. (The child will) presently come down.

Pan Chang Chan
Placenta Intestine Delivery
(*i.e.*, Wound Umbilical Cord Delivery)

(In) *pan chang chan* or wound umbilical cord delivery, the umbilical cord precedes the child. If the cord is not withdrawn in time, grind 49 seeds of Semen Ricini Communis (*Bi Ma Zi*) and apply them to the head. When the cord begins to withdraw, wash these off immediately; otherwise they do harm. Another method (is to) grind only 40 skinned seeds into a paste and apply this to the vertex. As soon as the cord begins to withdraw, wash this off (as well).

Nan Chan
Difficult Delivery

For difficult delivery (or) inability to bring forth the child due to failure of the joined bones to separate, administer ***Jia Wei Xiong Gui Tang*** (Added Flavors *Dang Gui* & Ligusticum Decoction) and after some time, (the child) will presently come down.

Rhizoma Ligustici Wallichii (*Xiao Chuan Xiong*), 1 *liang*
Radix Angelicae Sinensis (*Dang Gui*) 1 *liang*
Plastrum Praeparatum Testudinis (*Bai Gui Ban*), 1 piece, fried with wine
Crinis Carbonisatus (*Fu Ren Fa Hui*), 1 handful

Boil in 1 cup of water down to 7/10 (of a cup) and take.

Si Chan
Dead (Fetus) Delivery

Si chan or dead delivery means fetal death within the abdomen. If the tongue of the mother is green-blue and black, the fetus is dead. (In that case,) boil 1 *ji* of *Ping Wei San* (Level the Stomach Powder)[3] in a mixture of 1 cup of water and 1 cup of wine down to 8/10. Place this in *Pu Xiao Jian*[4] and continue to boil. Take this and (the dead fetus) will presently come down. Using children's urine is also good. Afterwards, use supplementing prescriptions to balance and regulate.

Xia Tai
Descending the Fetal (Placenta)

In case the fetal placenta does not descend, use 1 *ji* of *Shi Xiao San* (Laugh-exciting Powder) with warm wine, 1 *ji* of *Yi Mu Wan* (Boost the Mother Pill), 1 *ji* of *Sheng Hua Tang* (Generating & Transforming Decoction) with 1 *qian* of ash of Cornu Cervi Parvum (*Lu Jiao Hui*) mixed in, or provoke vomiting by means of putting the hair of the birthing woman in her mouth and the placenta will be exited or discharged presently. Inability to bring the placenta forth due to qi vacuity must be accompanied by abdominal distention and pain. Use only ***Sheng Hua Tang***:

Radix Angelicae Sinensis (*Quan Dang Gui*), 1 *liang*
Rhizoma Ligustici Wallichii (*Chuan Xiong*), 3 *qian*
Rhizoma Atractylodis Macrocephalae (*Bai Zhu*), 1 *qian*

---

3 The ingredients are given below under the next disease category.

4 The ingredients of this formula are given below under *Shi Xiao San* (Laugh-exciting Powder) in the next disease category.

Rhizoma Cyperi Rotundi (*Xiang Fu*), 1 *qian*

Decoct in water and take. It is even better if 3 *qian* of Radix Panacis Ginseng (*Ren Shen*) is added.

Another method (is to) grind Semen Ricini Communis (*Bi Ma Zi*), 2 *liang*, and Realgar (*Xiong Huang*), 2 *qian*, into a paste and apply this to *Yong Quan* (Ki 1) on the soles (of the feet). Immediately (after) the placenta has dropped, wash this off.

Ping Wei San (Level the Stomach Powder)

Rhizoma Atractylodis (*Nan Cang Zhu*), soaked in rice water & stir-fried
Cortex Magnoliae Officinalis (*Hou Po*), stir-fried with ginger
Pericarpium Citri Reticulatae (*Chen Pi*)
Radix Praeparatus Glycyrrhizae (*Zhi Gan Cao*)

Powder coarsely 2 *qian* of each (of the above) and decoct in either water or wine. After (the mixture) is boiled down to the desired degree, put in 2 *qian* of *Pu Xiao* and continue boiling for 1 minute. To be taken warm.

Shi Xiao San (Laugh-exciting Powder)

Feces Trogopterori Seu Pteromi (*Wu Ling Zhi*)
Pollen Typhae (*Pu Huang*)

Grind fine. Take 3 *qian* (once, chased) down with warm wine.

Duan Qi
Severing the Navel (*i.e.*, the Umbilical Cord)

Severing the umbilical cord is certainly best accomplished by biting through a cloth wrapping the cord. In cold weather or in case of difficult delivery where the mother and child are (both) fatigued, it is proper to slowly burn it asunder with a lighted paper scroll infused with hemp oil in order to assist the original qi. Even if the child is dead, sending warm qi into the umbilicus may bring back life in many cases. In any event, do not cut the cord with a knife.

Hua Tai San (Slippery Fetus Powder) [To make delivery easy, take several *ji* (of this powder) in the month before delivery.]

Radix Angelicae Sinensis (*Dang Gui*), 3-5 *qian*
Rhizoma Ligustici Wallichii (*Chuan Xiong*), 5-7 *qian*
Cortex Eucommiae Ulmoidis (*Du Zhong*), 2 *qian*
Radix Coquitus Rehmanniae (*Shu Di*), 3 *qian*
Fructus Citri Seu Ponciri (*Zhi Qiao*), 7 *fen*
Radix Dioscoreae Oppositae (*Shan Yao*), 2 *qian*

Boil in 2 cups of water down to 8/10 and take warm before meals. For a woman with qi vacuity and a weak body or constitution, add Radix Panacis Ginseng (*Ren Shen*) and Rhizoma Atractylodis Macrocephalae (*Bai Zhu*), the amount depending on necessity. In case of fecal stoppage with solid stools, add 2 *qian* of Radix Achyranthis Bidentatae (*Niu Xi*).

Zhi Chan Mi Yan Liang Fang (Secret, Proven, Efficacious Formula for Treating Birthing)

(This formula) treats transverse birth or inverted delivery when labor has lasted several days but the child is not yet brought forth. One *ji* will bring down (the child). In case of sudden stirring of the fetus before mature, one *ji* will calm it. Administering one *ji* towards delivery ensures safety. (This formula) is particularly effective in treating fetal death within the abdomen as well as miscarriage injury of the fetus and absence of breast milk. Take once (and) it will effect a perfect recovery.

Radix Angelicae Sinensis (*Quan Dang Gui*)
Rhizoma Ligustici Wallichii (*Chuan Xiong*), both 1.5 *qian*
Bulbus Fritillariae Cirrhosae (*Chuan Bei Mu*), 1 *qian*, cored
Herba Seu Flos Schizonepetae Tenuifoliae (*Jing Jie Sui*)
Radix Astragali Seu Hedysari (*Huang Qi*), both 8 *fen*
Cortex Magnoliae Officinalis (*Hou Po*), stir-fried with ginger
Folium Artemisiae Argyii (*Qi Ai*)
Flos Carthami Tinctorii (*Hong Hua*), 7 *fen* for the above three
Semen Cuscutae (*Tu Si Zi*), 1.2 *qian*
Radix Glycyrrhizae (*Gan Cao*), 5 *fen*
Radix Et Rhizoma Notopterygii (*Qiang Huo*), 6 *fen*, stir-fried with wheat flour
Fructus Citri Seu Ponciri (*Zhi Qiao*), 6 *fen*, stir-fried with wheat flour
Radix Albus Paeoniae Lactiflorae (*Bai Shao*), 1.2 *qian*, excluded in winter

Of these 13 ingredients, 12 are used (at any one time) in practice and the formula does not allow for (any other) modification. To calm the fetus, subtract Flos Carthami Tinctorii. To hasten birth, subtract Folium Artemisiae Argyii. (Boil) in 1 1/2 cups of well water and take warm with 3 slices of ginger as conductor. (Then) the dregs are to be boiled in 1 cup of water down to 1/2 and the decoction is to be taken warm. If no effect is brought, boil (the dregs) in 1 cup of water down to half again. After this is taken, effect will surely be achieved. There is no need to administer a second *ji*.

Cui Sheng Tu Nao Wan (Hasten Birth *Tu Nao* Pill) [Offers miraculous effect for transverse birth and inverted delivery.]

Rabbit brains (*Tu Nao*), killed in the 12th month, 1 head
Flos Syzygii Aromatici (*Mu Ding Xiang*), 1 piece
Gummum Olibani (*Ru Xiang*), 1 *qian*, ground separately
Secretio Moschi Moschiferi (*She Xiang*), 1 *fen*

Make into pills the size of gorgon fruit, dry in the shade, and seal tightly. When necessary, take 1 pill with warm wine.

Duo Ming Dan (Snatching Back Life Elixir)

At the point of delivery, in case of up-turned eyes, clenched jaw, a black facial complexion, green-blue lips, and foaming at the mouth, life is at stake. If the facial complexion is tinged with faint red, the fetus will die and the mother survive. Immediately administer:

Pellis Serpentis (*She Tui*), burnt without preserving (its) nature
Bombyx Mori (*Can Gu Zi*), burnt without preserving (its) nature
Crinis Carbonisatus (*Fa Hui*), 1 *qian*
Gummum Olibani (*Ru Xiang*), 5 *fen*

Powder fine (and chase) down with wine.

Jia Wei Xong Gui Tang (Added Flavors *Dang Gui* & Ligusticum Decoction) [Treats non-contraction and postpartum non-closure of the *zi gong* or uterus.]

Radix Panacis Ginseng (*Ren Shen*), 2 *qian*
Radix Astragali Seu Hedysari (*Huang Qi*), 1 *qian*
Radix Angelicae Sinensis (*Dang Gui*), 2 *qian*
Rhizoma Cimicifugae (*Sheng Ma*), 8 *fen*

Rhizoma Ligustici Wallichii (*Chuan Xiong*), 1 *qian*
Radix Praeparatus Glycyrrhizae (*Zhi Gan Cao*), 4 *fen*
Fructus Schizandrae Chinensis (*Wu Wei Zi*), 15 pieces

If the uterus still refuses to contract, add 8 *fen* of Rhizoma Pinelliae Ternatae (*Ban Xia*) and 8 *fen* of Radix Albus Paeoniae Lactiflorae (*Bai Shao*) stir-fried with wine.

Xin Chan Zhi Fa
Treatment Methods for the Newly Birthed

First, administer 2 *ji* of *Sheng Hua Tang* in succession. If the woman was weak before delivery, manifests a critical or hot condition, or (in case of) miscarriage, administer this decoction till recovery. (In those cases,) the number of *ji* may be unlimited. In case of overtaxation during labor or profuse bleeding deserting the body, add 3-4 *qian* of Radix Panacis Ginseng (*Ren Shen*). Administering this decoction at short intervals will ensure safety. In case of distressed, rapid breathing, also add Radix Panacis Ginseng. Addition of Radix Panacis Ginseng to this decoction prevents blood lumps from stagnation. It is wrong not to use Radix Panacis Ginseng thinking that it is a supplementing (medicinal). Some people exclude Radix Angelicae Sinensis (*Dang Gui*) when treating postpartum cases. This view is extremely one-sided. This formula is well designed and free from imperfection. It works unfailingly. People who treat postpartum cases with *Si Wu Tang* (Four Ingredient Decoction) are quite wrong, for Radix Coquitus Rehmanniae (*Di Huang*), (being) cold in nature, stagnates the blood, while Radix Albus Paeoniae Lactiflorae (*Shao Yao*), slightly sour, offers no supplementation but attacks and injures the qi.

Chan Hou Yong Yao Shi Wu
Ten Mistakes in Using Medicinals Postpartum

1. Even though the qi is unsoothed, it is a mistake to use qi-consuming or qi-normalizing medicinals which only make stuffiness and oppression worse. (Consequently,) Pericarpium Citri Reticulatae (*Chen Pi*) is limited to 5 *fen*. Fructus Immaturus Citri Seu Ponciri (*Zhi Shi*) and Cortex Magnoliae Officinalis (*Hou Po*) are contraindicated.

2. Even though there is injury of the qi, it is a mistake to use abducting dispersion which only injures stomach qi even possibly to the extent of inability to take in food. (Consequently,) Fructus Citri Seu Ponciri (*Zhi Qiao*), Radix Et Rhizoma Rhei (*Da Huang*), Rhizoma Curcumae Zedoariae (*Peng E Zhu*), Rhizoma Sparganii (*San Leng*), Massa Medica Fermentata (*Shen Qu*), and Cortex Magnoliae Officinalis (*Hou Po*) are contraindicated.

3. Even though the body is hot, it is a mistake to use cold and cooling (medicinals) which will, unavoidably, damage the stomach and increase heat. (Consequently,) Radix Scutellariae Baicalensis (*Huang Qin*), Rhizoma Coptidis Chinensis (*Huang Lian*), Fructus Gardeniae Jasminoidis (*Zhi Zi*), Cortex Phellodendri (*Huang Bai*), Rhizoma Cimicifugae (*Sheng Ma*), and Radix Bupleuri (*Chai Hu*) are contraindicated.

4. Even though one has administered *Sheng Hua Tang* recently, no Radix Panacis Ginseng (*Ren Shen*), Radix Astragali Seu Hedysari (*Huang Qi*), or Rhizoma Atractylodis Macrocephalae (*Bai Zhu*) should be taken as long as (blood) lump pain still lingers.

5. Do not use Radix Coquitus Rehmanniae (*Di Huang*) since it stagnates the lochia.

6. To dissipate (blood) lumps, do not use Fructus Citri Seu Ponciri (*Zhi Qiao*), Radix Achyranthis Bidentatae (*Niu Xi*), or Fructus Immaturus Citri Seu Ponciri (*Zhi Shi*).

7. In case of constipation, do not use Radix Et Rhizoma Rhei (*Da Huang*) or Mirabilitum (*Mang Xiao*).

8. To move (blood) lumps, do not use Lignum Sappanis (*Su Mu*), Rhizoma Sparganii (*San Leng*), or Rhizoma Curcumae Zedoariae (*Peng E Zhu*). Radix Albus Paeoniae Lactiflorae (*Bai Shao*) should not be used since it is capable of attacking the qi.

9. Do not use *Shan Zha Tang* (Crataegus Decoction)[5] to attack (blood) lumps or settle pain. It will, on the contrary, injure the new blood.

10. Do not administer without warrant *Ji Kun Dan* (Rescue Females Elixir)[6] to descend the fetus (*tai*, or) descend the placenta (*bao*).

In the treatment of various critical postpartum conditions, it is proper to administer *Sheng Hua Tang* at short intervals with appropriate additions and deletions according to the signs.

Chan Hou Han Re
Postpartum Cold (&) Heat

Shortly after delivery, because both *ying* and *wei* are vacuous, (women) are liable to cold and heat as well as body and abdominal pain. It is absolutely impermissible to prescribe

---

5 This formula is composed of Fructus Crataegi (*Shan Zha*), Massa Medica Fermentata (*Shen Qu*), and stir-fried Fructus Germinatus Hordei Vulgaris (*Mai Ya*).

6 Identification of the ingredients of this formula unknown.

effusing and dissipating formulas without warrant. One should prescribe *Sheng Hua Tang* as the basis with a small amount of effusing agents as assistants. After delivery, because the spleen is vacuous and liable to food stagnation, body heat or a generalized fever may result. Whenever they see body heat, people nowadays tend to ascribe this to external invasion and rashly use diaphoresis. This accelerates collapse tremendously. It is proper (instead) to add spleen-supporting and food-dispersing medicinals to *Sheng Hua Tang.* Generally speaking, after delivery, it is necessary to supplement first the blood and then the qi.

(However,) it is not wise to only use Radix Panacis Ginseng (*Ren Shen*) and Radix Astragali Seu Hedysari (*Huang Qi*) to solely supplement the qi. To supplement postpartum vacuity, use Radix Panacis Ginseng, Radix Astragali Seu Hedysari, Rhizoma Ligustici Wallichii (*Chuan Xiong*), Radix Angelicae Sinensis (*Dang Gui*), Rhizoma Atractylodis Macrocephalae (*Bai Zhu*), Pericarpium Citri Reticulatae (*Chen Pi*), and Radix Praeparatus Glycyrrhizae (*Zhi Gan Cao*).

In case of slight heat, use bland percolators such as Sclerotium Poriae Cocoris (*Fu Ling*) and the heat will disappear by itself. In case of severe (heat), add Rhizoma Desiccata Zingiberis (*Gan Jiang*). It may be questioned what good it is using Rhizoma Zingiberis in the presence of great heat. The answer is that it is not a replete heat but a heat generated by yin vacuity in the interior. Rhizoma Desiccata Zingiberis is able not only to enter the lung phase or *fei fen* to disinhibit the lung qi but also to enter the liver phase (*gan fen*) to conduct the various medicinals to generate the blood. It must be used, however, in combination with yin and blood medicinals. Postpartum aversion to cold with fever is necessarily ascribed to malign blood (*e xue*) if abdominal pain is present but not so if abdominal pain is absent.

Postpartum cold and heat and deviated eyes and mouth are due to severe vacuity of the qi and blood. Thus, great supplementation should mainly be used. If the pulse on the left hand is insufficient, blood-supplementing medicinals should be used more than qi-supplementing medicinals. (However,) if the pulse on the right hand is insufficient, more medicinals should be used to supplement the qi than to supplement the blood. Do not, at any rate, use effusing, dissipating formulas such as *Xiao Xu Ming Tang* (Minor Reinforce Life).[7]

Tai Qian Huan Shang Han Yi Zheng Nue Yi Duo Tai Deng Zheng
Before Birth Contraction of Cold Injury, Epidemic Disease, Malaria, Miscarriage, etc.[8]

If there is cold injury before delivery, epidemic disease, or malaria, enduring heat will inevitably result in miscarriage. After miscarriage, heat will increase because it consumes yin/blood and because abortion is followed by blood loss. The practitioner must guard against misusing *Zhi Zi Chi Tang* (Gardenia & Fermented Soybean Decoction)[9] or such medicinals as Radix Bupleuri (*Chai Hu*), Radix Scutellariae Baicalensis

---

7 This formula is composed of Herba Ephedrae Chinensis (*Ma Huang*), 1 *liang;* Ramulus Cinnamomi (*Gui Zhi*), 1 *liang;* Rhizoma Ligustici Wallichii (*Chuan Xiong*), 1 *liang;* Radix Panacis Ginseng (*Ren Shen*), 1 *liang;* Radix Albus Paeoniae Lactiflorae (*Shao Yao*), 1 *liang;* Semen Pruni Armeniacae (*Xing Ren*), 1 *liang;* Radix Scutellariae Baicalensis (*Huang Qin*), 1 *liang;* Radix Stephaniae Tetrandrae (*Fang Ji*), 1 *liang;* Radix Glycyrrhizae (*Gan Cao*), 1 *liang;* Radix Praeparatus Aconiti Carmichaeli (*Fu Zi*), 1 piece; Radix Ledebouriellae Sesloidis (*Fang Feng*), 1.5 *liang;* Rhizoma Recens Zingiberis (*Sheng Jiang*).

8 The *huan* in this title is very probably a misprint.

9 This formula is composed of Fructus Gardeniae Jasminoidis (*Zhi Zi*), 14 pieces, and Semen Praeparatus Sojae (*Dou Chi*), 4 *he*, decocted in water.

(*Huang Qin*), Rhizoma Coptidis Chinensis (*Huang Lian*), and Cortex Phellodendri (*Huang Bai*) due to miscalculation of the fact that cold injury or epidemic disease have not yet been eliminated. Even in case of intermittent tidal fever, constipation, and urine stoppage, *Wu Ling (San)* (Five *Ling* Powder)[10], *Cheng Qi (Tang,* Qi-Supporting Decoction), or the like is absolutely prohibited. It is necessary to subordinate (the treatment of) evils to the treatment of postpartum conditions and to apply great supplementation of the qi and blood by administering *Sheng Hua Tang* at short intervals. In case of form desertion (*ti tuo*) and qi desertion, add *Sheng Mai San* (Generate the Pulse Powder)[11] to prevent blood dizziness. Rhizoma Ligustici Wallichii (*Chuan Xiong*) is acrid in flavor and capable of dissipating, while Rhizoma Desiccata Zingiberis (*Gan Jiang*) is able to eliminate vacuity fire. Therefore, even in case of constipation, vexing thirst, etc., administer merely a great deal of *Sheng Hua Tang* and fluids will naturally be generated and urination and defecation freed. If cold formulas are used for heat (postpartum), central qi is made (even) more vacuous. (This is) a serious fault.

---

10 This formula consists of Rhizoma Atractylodis (*Cang Zhu)*, 18 *zhu;* Sclerotium Polypori Umbellati (*Zhu Ling*), 18 *zhu;* Sclerotium Poriae Cocoris (*Fu Ling*), 18 *zhu;* Rhizoma Alismatis (*Ze Xie*), 1 *liang* 6 *zhu;* and Ramulus Cinnamomi (*Gui Zhi*), 0.5 *liang*. 1 *zhu* = 1/24 *liang*.

11 The ingredients of this formula include Tuber Ophiopogonis Japonicae (*Mai Dong*), 3 *qian;* Fructus Schizandrae Chinensis (*Wu Wei Zi*), 2 *qian;* and Radix Panacis Ginseng (*Ren Shen*), 5 *qian*.

Chapter 3

Chan Hou Zhu Zheng Zhi Fa
Treatment Methods for Various Postpartum Conditions

Xue Kuai
Blood Clots

(To treat) this disorder, do not blindly adhere to the ancient formulas. Indiscreet use of Lignum Sappanis (*Su Mu*), Rhizoma Curcumae Zedoariae (*Peng E Zhu*), and Rhizoma Sparganii (*San Leng*) is to take lightly others' lives. All the blood-dissipating formulas and blood-cracking medicinals are prohibited. Moderate as Fructus Crataegi (*Shan Zha*) is, it can take life and, therefore, should not be used without warrant. The only divine formula to treat blood clots is *Sheng Hua Tang*.

Sheng Hua Tang (Generating & Transforming Decoction)[Original formula]

Radix Angelicae Sinensis (*Dang Gui*), 8 *qian*
Rhizoma Ligustici Wallichii (*Chuan Xiong*), 3 *qian*
Semen Pruni Persicae (*Tao Ren*), 14 pieces, skinned, tip-nipped, (&) ground
Rhizoma Carbonisata Zingiberis (*Hei Jiang*), 5 *fen*
Radix Praeparatus Glycyrrhizae (*Zhi Gan Cao*), 5 *fen*

Decoct in equal amount of Shaoxing wine and child's urine and take.

Another (therapy): Take *Yi Mu Wan* (Boost the Mother Pill) and 1 *qian* of ash of Cornu Cervi Parvum (*Lu Jiao Hui*) with *Sheng Hua Tang*. As external treatment, heat cloths by fire to warm the place of the painful lump. This should be done even during the time of Great Heat.[1] Be sure not to unjustifiably ascribe stupor and inversion due to non-movement of the qi to malign blood rushing upon the heart. It is desirable to use only *Sheng Hua Tang*. There is a popular belief that Radix Rehmanniae (*Sheng Di*) and Radix Achyranthis Bidentatae (*Niu Xi*) move the blood, Rhizoma Sparganii (*San Leng*) and Rhizoma Curcumae Zedoariae (*E Zhu*) vanquish the blood, Fructus Crataegi (*Shan Zha*) and granulated sugar (*Sha Tang*) dissipate lumps, and that Folium Artemisiae Argyii (*Qi Ai*) and Fructus Zanthoxyli Bungeani wine (*Jiao Jiu*) settle pain. On the contrary, (during the puerperium,) they cause such disorders as clouding and dizziness and, therefore, should not be introduced without warrant. If the pain feels better after two, three, or four days and can be relieved by kneading, this is vacuity pain. It is appropriate to administer *Jia Shen Sheng Hua Tang* (Added Ginseng Generating & Transforming Decoction).

If bound or knotted lumps give serious pain within seven days (of delivery), possibly owing to cold and cool food, add 8 *fen* [3 *fen* in a variant edition] of Cortex Cinnamomi (*Rou Gui*) to *Sheng Hua Tang*. Do not add Radix Panacis Ginseng (*Ren Shen*) or Radix Astragali Seu Hedysari (*Huang Qi*) before these blood lumps are eliminated. Otherwise, the pain will become enduring. In sum, be sure not to use harshly disinhibiting medicinals, do not take much wine (made from) Rhizoma

---

1 This is one of the 14-day solar periods of the Chinese farmer's almanac.

Zingiberis (*Jiang*), Fructus Zanthoxyli Bungeani (*Jiao*), or Folium Artemisiae Argyii (*Ai*), but frequently take *Sheng Hua Tang* to move the qi and assist the blood. And, as external treatment, use heated clothes to warm the abdomen. Similarly, using Flos Carthami Tinctorii (*Hong Hua*) to move and Lignum Sappanis (*Su Mu*) and Radix Achyranthis Bidentatae (*Niu Xi*) to attack leads to harm. In case of fetal qi distention, use of Radix Linderae Strychnifoliae (*Wu Yao*) and Rhizoma Cyperi Rotundi (*Xiang Fu*) to normalize (the qi); Fructus Citri Seu Ponciri (*Zhi Qiao*) and Cortex Magnoliae Officinalis (*Hou Po*) to soothe (the qi); in serious cases, Pericarpium Viridis Citri Reticulatae (*Qing Pi*), Fructus Immaturus Citri Seu Ponciri (*Zhi Shi*), Fructus Perillae Frutescentis (*Su Zi*) to downbear qi and stabilize dyspnea; and Radix Scutellariae Baicalensis (*Huang Qin*), Rhizoma Coptidis Chinensis (*Huang Lian*), Fructus Gardeniae Jasminoidis (*Zhi Zi*), and Cortex Phellodendri (*Huang Bai*) to abate heat and eliminate vexation (all cause harm). As to still more serious blood binding, inappropriately using *Cheng Qi Tang* to purge or precipitate will make this binding (even) more serious. (Likewise,) in case of profuse sweating with short, inhibited urination, inappropriate use of *Wu Ling San* to free flow will make this stoppage (even) more serious. Far from doing good, these bring harm.

Generally speaking, after the child is delivered, in case of retention of blood still giving pain half a month later, toxic swelling rising 1 *cun* or so in height, or body heat or generalized fever with reduced appetite and severe fatigue, there is no other choice but to administer *Sheng Hua Tang* with the addition of Rhizoma Sparganii (*San Leng*), Rhizoma Curcumae Zedoariae (*Peng E Zhu*), Cortex Cinnamomi (*Rou Gui*), and the like so as to attack and supplement simultaneously. Then the (blood) lump will disappear of itself. In case of severe vacuity with diminished food intake and diarrhea, take only this decoction to settle pain. It is, in addition, capable of fortifying the spleen and stomach, promoting digestion and stopping diarrhea. Then administer the *Xiao Kuai Tang* (Dissipating Lump Decoction).[2]

Jia Wei Sheng Hua Tang (Added Flavors Generating & Transforming Decoction) [Treats persisting blood lump. Do not administer till half a month after (delivery).]

Rhizoma Ligustici Wallichii (*Chuan Xiong*), 1 *qian*
Radix Angelicae Sinensis (*Dang Gui*), 3 *qian*
Rhizoma Zingiberis (*Rou Jiang*), 4 *fen*
Semen Pruni Persicae (*Tao Ren*), 15 pieces
Rhizoma Sparganii (*San Leng*), stir-fried with vinegar, 6 fen
Rhizoma Corydalis Yanhusuo (*Yuan Hu*), 6 *fen*
Cortex Cinnamomi (*Rou Gui*), 6 *fen*
Radix Praeparatus Glycyrrhizae (*Zhi Gan Cao*), 4 *fen*

Xue Yun
Blood Dizziness

Following delivery, black flowery vision, spinning head, clouding, dizziness, and loss of consciousness are caused by 1) qi exhaustion and spirit clouding due to severe fatigue; 2) impending expiration of qi due to great desertion of blood; 3) spirit failing to keep (to its abode) due to phlegm fire taking advantage of qi vacuity. (For these,) 2 or 3 *ji* of *Sheng Hua Tang* should be administered immediately. As an external treatment, cut Bulbus Allii Tuberosi (*Jiu Cai*) fine, put it in a bottle with a (small) opening, pour in 2 cups of boiling vinegar, and immediately let (the steam) penetrate the nose of the birthing

2 This probably does not refer so much to a specific formula as to a class of formulas which disperse glomus, lumps, etc. In the following section on blood dizziness, there are given a number of such formulas.

mother. Then she will presently come to. It is a grave mistake if, out of a blind belief in the *gu fang* or ancient formulas, (one) indiscreetly uses blood-dissipating medicinals on the assumption of malign blood surging into the heart or uses a non-supplementing, dispersing, downbearing formula on the assumption of epidemic fire.

In case of clouding inversion with clenched teeth, boil up some *Sheng Hua Tang* immediately, pry the teeth, probe the throat with a goose quill, and then pour down the decoction with a (small) wine cup. If the abdomen gets warmer as the decoction is being poured down, (continue the administration) without regard to the number of *ji*. As an external treatment, press and rub the patient through thin clothes from the heart down to the abdomen with a warm hand which should be heated by fire frequently. In one or two watches, after 4 *ji* of the decoction are finished, the spirit will become clear. Now slow down the administration of the decoction and then feed a little porridge. When 10 *ji* are finished, (the patient is) safe. Therefore, in case of such an attack, pour (down the throat) the decoction promptly and keep (the patient) warm by fire. It is not permitted to give up (the patient) and abandon rescue efforts. In winter months, if the woman's body cannot be kept warm, there will be serious danger. Towards delivery, it is necessary to have *Sheng Hua Tang* prepared and weights from the steelyard or stones heated. After the child is delivered, take 2 or 3 *jis* in succession. In addition, dizziness can surely be prevented by performing the pouring of vinegar and Allium Tuberosum into a bottle method at the pillow of the birthing woman. What's more, after the child is delivered, the family should not take delight in the child to the neglect of the mother. Nor should the mother so indulge in the child as to forget her own fatigue, lie down upon finishing delivery, or get enraged so as to provoke qi counterflow. Any (of the above) may lead to *xue yun* or blood dizziness. Take care! Take care!

Jia Wei Sheng Hua Tang (Added Flavors Generating & Transforming Decoction [Treats the three types of blood dizziness]

Rhizoma Ligustici Wallichii (*Chuan Xiong*), 3 *qian*
Radix Angelicae Sinensis (*Dang Gui*), 6 *qian*
Rhizoma Carbonisata Zingiberis (*Hei Jiang*), 4 *fen*
Semen Pruni Persicae (*Tao Ren*), 10 pieces
Radix Praeparatus Glycyrrhizae (*Zhi Gan Cao*), 5 *fen*
Herba Seu Flos Schizonepetae Tenuifoliae (*Jing Jie*), 4 *fen*, char-fried
Fructus Zizyphi Jujubae (*Da Zao*)

Decoct in water and take. In case of dizziness either due to severe fatigue or due to profuse bleeding and qi desertion, it is proper to pour 2 *ji* (down the throat) instantly. In case of either form and complexion desertion or sweating desertion due to (copious) perspiration, administer 1 *ji* immediately with the addition of 3-4 *qian* of Radix Panacis Ginseng (*Ren Shen*) [4 *fen* of Cortex Cinnamomi (*Rou Gui*) in a variant edition]. Do not delay in any event administering Radix Panacis Ginseng on the grounds that it is a supplementing (medicinal). In case of dizziness due to phlegm fire taking advantage of vacuity to flame upward, add 4 *fen* of Exocarpium Citri Rubri (*Ju Hong*) to the formula. In case of severe vacuity, add 2 *qian* of Radix Panacis Ginseng. For a fat patient who is abundant in phlegm, add, in addition, 7 *fen* of Succus Bambusae (*Zhu Li*) and a little Succus Zingiberis (*Jiang Zhi*). In no case should a blood-cracking formula composed of Rhizoma Sparganii (*San Leng*), Rhizoma Curcumae Zedoariae (*E Zhu*,) or the like be employed. In case of severe lump pain, administer, in addition, *Yi Mu Wan* (Boost the Mother Pill), ash of Cornu Cervi Parvum

(*Lu Jiao Hui*), *Yuan Hu San* (Corydalis Powder)[3], or *Du Sheng San* (Unique Conquering Powder).[4] Of the above blood lump-dispersing formulas, take only one (of them) and the effect will be achieved. There is no need to change to another (half way). Emergency treatment should be performed in accordance with the conditions.

Jia Shen Sheng Hua Tang (Added Ginseng Generating & Transforming Decoction) [Treats postpartum dizziness with form and complexion desertion or with sweating desertion due to copious perspiration]

Radix Panacis Ginseng (*Ren Shen*), 3 *qian*, may be increased to 5 *qian* in some cases
Rhizoma Ligustici Wallichii (*Chuan Xiong*), 2 *qian*
Radix Angelicae Sinensis (*Dang Gui*), 5 *qian*
Radix Praeparatus Glycyrrhizae (*Zhi Gan Cao*), 4 *fen*
Semen Pruni Persicae (*Tao Ren*), 10 pieces
Rhizoma Praeparata Zingiberis (*Pao Jiang*), 4 *fen*
Fructus Ziziphi Jujubae (*Da Zao*)

Decoct in water and take.

---

3 This formula is composed of Rhizoma Corydalis Yanhusuo (*Yuan Hu*), Radix Angelicae Sinensis (*Dang Gui*), Pollen Typhae (*Pu Huang*), Radix Rubrus Paeoniae Lactiflorae (*Chi Shao*), Cortex Cinnamomi (*Guan Gui*), each 1 *qian*; Rhizoma Curcumae (*Jiang Huang*), Radix Saussureae Seu Vladimiriae (*Mu Xiang*), Gummum Olibani (*Ru Xiang*), Myrrha (*Mo Yao*), each 7 *fen*; Radix Praeparatus Glycyrrhizae (*Zhi Gan Cao*), 5 *fen*; and Rhizoma Recens Zingiberis (*Sheng Jiang*), 3 slices.

4 This is composed of Radix Angelicae Duhuo (*Du Huo*), Cortex Radix Lycii (*Di Gu Pi*), Herba Cum Radice Asari Sieboldi (*Xi Xin*), Rhizoma Ligustici Wallichii (*Chuan Xiong*), Flos Chrysanthemi Morifolii (*Ju Hua*), Radix Ledebouriellae Sesloidis (*Fang Feng*), Radix Praeparatus Glycyrrhizae (*Zhi Gan Cao*), all in equal amounts.

In case of pulse desertion and form desertion, which are conditions of impending expiration, there is no other choice but to administer this formula with 4-5 *qian* of Radix Panacis Ginseng (*Ren Shen*) added. Pour the decoction (down the throat of the patient) at short intervals. In case of postpartum profuse bleeding and blood dizziness with profuse sweating, it is appropriate to administer this formula. In case of absence of sweating and no desertion, administer only the primary formula with no need of adding Radix Panacis Ginseng. If the *chi* or foot pulse on the left deserts, also add Radix Panacis Ginseng. This formula can be used to treat various postpartum critical and acute conditions. In a day and night, it is necessary to take 3-4 *ji*. If it is taken as in an ordinary case, how can it reinforce the qi and blood which are already bordering on expiration or rescue critical or acute transmuted conditions? One or two days after delivery, if the birthing woman with blood lump pain not yet relieved has qi and blood vacuity desertion with dizziness, inversion, profuse sweating, form desertion with the qi from the mouth gradually getting cooler and constant vexing thirst, or rapid dyspneic breathing, administer the *Jia Shen Sheng Hua Tang* as a first-aid measure irrespective of the presence of the lump pain. After the condition abates a little, it is (then) necessary to subtract Radix Panacis Ginseng and continue administering (plain) *Sheng Hua Tang*.

Methods of addition and subtraction: In case of severe lump pain, add 7 *fen* Cortex Cinnamomi (*Rou Gui*). In case of thirst, add 1 *qian* of Tuber Ophiopogonis Japonicae (*Mai Dong*) and 10 pieces of Fructus Schizandrae Chinensis (*Wu Wei*). In case of profuse sweating, add 1 *qian* of Radix Ephedrae Chinensis (*Ma Huang Geng*). But, to stop sweating in the absence of blood lump pain, add 1 *qian* of Radix Praeparatus Astragali Seu Hedysari (*Zhi Huang Qi*) instead. In case of cereal flour (type) food injury, add 1 *qian* of stir-fried Massa Medica Fermentata

(*Shen Qu*) and 5 *fen* of stir-fried Fructus Germinatus Hordei Vulgaris (*Mai Ya*). In case of meat type food injury, add 5 pieces of Fructus Crataegi (*Shan Zha*) and 4 *qian* of stir-fried Fructus Seu Semen Amomi (*Sha Ren*).

Ni Zheng
Inversion Condition

In the course of delivery, (some) women overexert themselves (with) taxation and fatigue injuring the spleen. As a result, there occurs inversion with counterflow chilling (of the limbs). Qi ascends to fill up the chest, the pulse departs, and form deserts. There is no other choice but to greatly supplement. How can several *qian* of Rhizoma Ligustici Wallichii (*Chuan Xiong*) or Radix Angelicae Sinensis (*Dang Gui*) (be expected to succeed in) recovering yang to restore the spirit? It is necessary to use *Jia Shen Sheng Hua Tang* (Added Ginseng Generating & Transforming Decoction) with a double amount of Radix Panacis Ginseng (*Ren Shen*). Two *ji* taken, qi and blood become effulgent, the spirit generates by itself, and inversion comes to an end by itself. Should thirst arise following the administration, *Sheng Mai San* (Generating the Pulse Powder) and *Du Shen (Tang,* Solitary Ginseng Decoction) can be drunk as tea to rescue the viscera from dryness. If counterflow chilling of the limbs is accompanied by yin patterns of diarrhea and quasi-cold injury, it is hardly possible to use *Si Ni Tang* (Four Counterflows Decoction). It is necessary to use *Sheng Hua Tang* with a double amount of Radix Panacis Ginseng (*Ren Shen*) and a slice of Radix Praeparatus Aconiti Carmichaeli (*Fu Zi*) to recover yang and stop counterflow as well as to bring into play the strength of the Radix Panacis Ginseng and Radix Angelicae Sinensis. Two formulas are given below (for use) before and after.

Jia Shen Sheng Hua Tang (Added Ginseng Generating & Transforming Decoction) [Treats postpartum inversion. Before lump pain is relieved, do not add Radix Astragali Seu Hedysari (*Huang Qi*) or Rhizoma Atractylodis Macrocephalae (*Bai Zhu*).]

Rhizoma Ligustici Wallichii (*Chuan Xiong*), 2 *qian*
Radix Angelicae Sinensis (*Dang Gui*), 4 *qian*
Radix Praeparatus Glycyrrhizae (*Zhi Gan Cao*), 5 *fen*
Rhizoma Praeparata Zingiberis (*Pao Jiang*), 4 *fen* [charred in a variant edition]
Semen Pruni Persicae (*Tao Ren*), 10 pieces, skinned, tip-nipped, (&) ground
Radix Panacis Ginseng (*Ren Shen*), 2 *qian*
Fructus Zizyphi Jujubae (*Zao*)

Decoct in water. Administer 2 *ji*.

Zi Rong Yi Qi Fu Shen Tang (Enrich Construction, Boost the Qi, & Restore the Spirit Decoction) [Treats postpartum inversion. Administer after making sure that lump pain is already relieved.]

Radix Panacis Ginseng (*Ren Shen*), 3 *qian*
Radix Astragali Seu Hedysari (*Huang Qi*), 1 *qian*, stir-fried with honey
Rhizoma Atractylodis Macrocephalae (*Bai Zhu*), 1 *qian*, stir-fried with earth
Radix Angelicae Sinensis (*Dang Gui*), 3 *qian*
Radix Praeparatus Glycyrrhizae (*Zhi Gan Cao*), 4 *fen*
Pericarpium Citri Reticulatae (*Chen Pi*), 4 *fen*
Fructus Schizandrae Chinensis (*Wu Wei*), 10 pieces
Rhizoma Ligustici Wallichii (*Chuan Xiong*), 1 *qian*
Radix Coquitus Rehmanniae (*Shu Di*), 1 *qian*
Fructus Germinatus Hordei Vulgaris (*Mai Ya*), 1 *qian*
Fructus Zizyphi Jujubae (*Zao*), 1 piece

Decoct in water and take.

In case of cold hands and feet, add 5 *fen* of Radix Praeparatus Aconiti Carmichaeli (*Fu Zi*). In case of profuse sweating, add 1 *qian* of Radix Ephedrae Chinensis (*Ma Huang Geng*) and 1 *qian* of cooked Semen Zizyphi Spinosae (*Zao Ren*). In case of confused vision and hearing, add Fructus Alpiniae Oxyphyllae (*Yi Zhi*), Semen Biotae Orientalis (*Bai Zi Ren*) and Arillus Euphoriae Longanae (*Long Yan Rou*). In case of solid stools, add 2 *qian* of Herba Cistanchis (*Rou Cong Rong*). Roughly speaking, postpartum dizziness and inversion are similar. Dizziness, however, happens in the process of labor and its signs are more acute than those of inversion. (For this,) it is proper to administer a number of *ji* of *Sheng Hua Tang* in quick succession. Then lumps will be transformed and blood will become effulgent, while the spirit will become clear and dizziness will be stopped. In case of additional signs of rapid dyspneic breathing and form desertion, it is absolutely necessary to add Radix Panacis Ginseng (*Ren Shen*) and Radix Astragali Seu Hedysari (*Huang Qi*). Inversion happens after delivery. *Sheng Hua Tang* with a double amount of Radix Panacis Ginseng is required to stop (this), to restore the spirit as well as supplement the qi and blood. (Inversion) cannot be cured by merely supplementing the qi and blood as said above. It should be understood that dizziness accompanies lump pain and, therefore, does not allow the introduction of Radix Astragali Seu Hedysari and Rhizoma Atractylodis Macrocephalae (*Bai Zhu*). In the case of inversion without lump pain, use of these two drugs and Radix Coquitus Rehmanniae (*Di Huang*) in combination goes without question.

Xue Beng
Profuse (Uterine) Bleeding

In case of enormous postpartum bleeding, (one should) distinguish if the blood is red or purple in color and determine if (the patient's) form and complexion are (indicative) of vacuity or repletion. If the blood is purple and contains clots, it is necessary to eliminate the vanquished blood whose stagnation and retention are the cause of pain. This should not be regarded as *xue beng* or profuse (uterine) bleeding. If the blood is bright red, this indicates inability (either) to generate blood due to the heart's being injured by fright, to store blood due to the liver's being injured by anger, or to govern blood due to the spleen's being injured by taxation. These are all (cases of blood) failing to return to the channels and should be treated as *xue beng* or profuse (uterine) bleeding.

First, administer a few *ji* of *Sheng Hua Tang* and supplementation will be naturally (realized) through moving (the blood). In case of form desertion, profuse sweating, and rapid dyspneic breathing, it is proper to administer several *ji*s of this decoction with a double amount of Radix Panacis Ginseng (*Ren Shen*) to boost the qi. It is not a (bleeding) that Folium Et Petriolus Carbonisatus Trachycarpi (*Zong Lu Hui*) is able to stop or if *xue beng* arises more than half a month after delivery, (then) the appropriate formula to treat these is *Sheng Ju Da Bu Tang* (Uplifting, Great Supplementing Decoction). Because this is a condition of extreme vacuity and (because,) after being taken, this decoction works steadily and temperantly, rapid effects cannot be expected. The various signs will not be abruptly eliminated until 20 *ji* have been administered.

Sheng Xue Zhi Beng Tang (Generate the Blood, Stop *Beng* Decoction) [Treats postpartum profuse (uterine) bleeding]

Rhizoma Ligustici Wallichii (*Chuan Xiong*), 1 *qian*
Radix Angelicae Sinensis (*Dang Gui*), 4 *qian*
Rhizoma Carbonisata Zingiberis (*Hei Jiang*), 4 *fen*
Radix Praeparatus Glycyrrhizae (*Zhi Gan Cao*), 5 *fen*
Semen Pruni Persicae (*Tao Ren*), 10 pieces
Herba Seu Flos Schizonepetae Tenuifoliae (*Jing Jie*), 5 *fen*, char-fried
Fructus Pruni Mume (*Wu Mei*), 5 *fen*, calcined to ash
Pollen Typhae (*Pu Huang*), 5 *fen*, stir-fried
Fructus Zizyphi Jujubae (*Zao*)

Decoct in water. (Eating) ginger, Szechuan pepper, hot, cold, and raw foods are prohibited.

[When using Herba Seu Flos Schizonepetae Tenuifoliae to stop *beng*, it must always be slightly blackened.]

In case of enormous running of bright red blood, (add) charred Herba Seu Flos Schizonepetae Tenuifoliae and Radix Angelicae (*Bai Zhi*), each 5 *fen*. In case of exhausted blood and vanquished form, add 3-4 *qian* of Radix Panacis Ginseng (*Ren Shen*). In case of profuse sweating and distressed rapid breathing, also add 3-4 *qian* of Radix Panacis Ginseng. In case of absence of sweating and non-desertion form but distressed rapid breathing, administer *Sheng Hua Tang* only. After taking a sufficient number of *ji*, the blood will become calm by itself. The charge that Radix Angelicae Sinensis and Rhizoma Ligustici Wallichii are merely capable of quickening the blood is categorically wrong.

Sheng Ju Da Bu Tang (Up-lifting, Greatly Supplementing Decoction) [Enriches the *ying* and boosts the qi. In case of lumps and stirring, administer the above formula only without using Radix Astragali Seu Hedysari (*Huang Qi*) or Rhizoma Atractylodis Macrocephalae (*Bai Zhu*).]

Radix Astragali Seu Hedysari (*Huang Qi*)
Rhizoma Atractylodis Macrocephalae (*Bai Zhu*)
Pericarpium Citri Reticulatae (*Chen Pi*), each 4 *fen*
Radix Panacis Ginseng (*Ren Shen*), 2 *qian*
Radix Praeparatus Glycyrrhizae (*Zhi Gan Cao*)
Rhizoma Cimicifugae (*Sheng Ma*), each 4 *fen*
Radix Angelicae Sinensis (*Dang Gui*)
Radix Coquitus Rehmanniae (*Shu Di*), each 2 *qian*
Tuber Ophiopogonis Japonicae (*Mai Dong*), 1 *qian*
Rhizoma Ligustici Wallichii (*Chuan Xiong*), 1 *qian*
Radix Angelicae (*Bai Zhi*), 4 *fen*
Rhizoma Coptidis Chinensis (*Huang Lian*), 3 *fen*, stir-fried
Herba Seu Flos Schizonepetae Tenuifoliae (*Jing Jie Sui*), 4 *fen*, char-fried

In case of profuse sweating, add 1 *qian* of Radix Ephedrae Chinensis (*Ma Huang Geng*) and a handful of Fructus Levis Tritici (*Fu Xiao Mai*). In case of constipation, add 1 *qian* of Herba Cistanchis (*Rou Cong Rong*) but never use Radix Et Rhizoma Rhei (*Da Huang*). In case of qi stagnation, add 3 *fen* of ground Radix Saussureae Seu Vladimiriae (*Mu Xiang*). In case of phlegm, add 6 *fen* of Bulbus Fritillariae Thunbergii (*Bei mu*) and a small amount of Succus Bambusae (*Zhi Li*) and Succus Zingiberis (*Jiang Zhi*). In case of cold coughing, add 10 seeds of Semen Pruni Armeniacae (*Xing Ren*), 5 *fen* of Radix Platycodi Grandiflori (*Jie Geng*), and 1 *qian* of Rhizoma Anemarrhenae (*Zhi Mu*). In case of fright, add Semen Zizyphi Spinosae (*Zao Ren*) and Semen Biotae Orientalis (*Bai Zi Ren*), 1 *qian* each. In case of grain (type) food injury, add Massa Medica Fermentata (*Shen Qu*) and Fructus Germinatus Hordei Vulgaris (*Mai Ya*), 1 *qian* each. In case of meat (type) food injury, add Fructus Crataegi (*Shan Zha*) and Fructus Seu Semen Amomi (*Sha Ren*), 8 *fen* each. To all (of these,) add Fructus Zizyphi Jujubae and decoct in water. In case of body heat, do not add Rhizoma Coptidis Chinensis (*Huang Lian*) or Cortex Phellodendri (*Huang*

Bai). In case of food injury or angry qi, do not exclusively use consuming, dissipating, non-supplementing medicinals. For *xue beng* in an old or vacuous person, *Sheng Ju Da Bu Tang* is the appropriate formula.

[In regards to an extreme vacuity condition, there is the instruction, "For body heat, do not use Rhizoma Coptidis Chinensis or Cortex Phellodendri." In a later place, under the entry *Fu Shen Tang* (Restore the Spirit Decoction), there is the instruction regarding that formula, "Use a small amount of Rhizoma Coptidis Chinensis as an assistant to downbear fire." If there is no fire to be downborne and since this formula consists of no hot medicinals, there is no need of a counterassistant and, hence, Rhizoma Coptidis Chinesis should not be used indiscriminately. Here, a most careful study is required. Also in the explanations above there is the instruction, "For cold coughing, it is proper to add Rhizoma Anemarrhenae." Since it is cold coughing, this drug should not be used unscrupulously. It is suspected that the word *han* or cold is a misprint in the original edition.]

Qi Duan Si Chuan
Shortness of Breath Similar to Asthma

Because of blood desertion and severe fatigue, qi may lose its support and, (therefore,) the breath may deviate from its normal pace. Some people suppose this is (due to) phlegm fire and thus mistakenly treat it with qi-dissipating, phlegm-transforming formulas. This puts the patient's life in peril. It is imperative to mainly and greatly supplement the blood. If there are lumps, do not use Radix Panacis Ginseng (*Ren Shen*), Radix Astragali Seu Hedysari (*Huang Qi*), or Rhizoma Atractylodis Macrocephalae (*Bai Zhu*). Only in the absence of lumps is the following formula applicable, (in which case,) Semen Pruni Persicae (*Tao Ren*) is left out and Radix Coquitus

Rehmanniae (*Shu Di*) and one slice of Radix Praeparatus Aconiti Carmichaeli (*Fu Zi*) are added. In case of cold feet, add 1 *qian* of cooked Radix Praeparatus Aconiti Carmichaeli (*Shu Fu Zi*) in addition to Radix Panacis Ginseng, Rhizoma Atractylodis Macrocephalae, and Pericarpium Citri Reticulatae (*Chen Pi*) and then continue with *Bu Qi Yang Rong Tang* (Supplement the Qi & Nurture the Construction Decoction).

Jia Shen Sheng Hua Tang (Added Ginseng Generating & Transforming Decoction) [Treats shortage of breath immediately following delivery. If there are lumps, do not add Radix Astragali Seu Hedysari or Rhizoma Atractylodis Macrocephalae.]

Rhizoma Ligustici Wallichii (*Chuan Xiong*), 2 *qian*
Radix Angelicae Sinensis (*Dang Gui*), 4 *qian*
Radix Praeparatus Glycyrrhizae (*Zhi Gan Cao*), 5 *fen*
Rhizoma Carbonisata Zingiberis (*Hei Jiang*), 4 *fen*
Semen Pruni Persicae (*Tao Ren*), 10 pieces, skinned, tip-nipped, (&) ground
Radix Panacis Ginseng (*Ren Shen*), 2 *qian*

Add 1 piece of Fructus Zizyphi Jujubae (*Da Zao*) as conductor. After 2-3 *ji* have been taken, change to the formula below.

Bu Qi Yang Rong Tang (Supplement the Qi, Nurture Construction Decoction) [Treats postpartum distressed short, rapid breathing. It is proper to administer this formula (only) in the absence of painful blood lumps.]

Radix Astragali Seu Hedysari (*Huang Qi*), 1 *qian*
Rhizoma Atractylodis Macrocephalae (*Bai Zhu*), 1 *qian*
Radix Angelicae Sinensis (*Dang Gui*), 4 *qian*
Radix Panacis Ginseng (*Ren Shen*), 3 *qian*
Pericarpium Citri Reticulatae (*Chen Pi*), 4 *fen*

Radix Praeparatus Glycyrrhizae (*Zhi Gan Cao*), 4 *fen*
Radix Coquitus Rehmanniae (*Shu Di*), 2 *qian*
Rhizoma Ligustici Wallichii (*Chuan Xiong*), 2 *qian*
Rhizoma Carbonisata Zingiberis (*Hei Jiang*), 4 *fen*

In case of cold hands and feet, add 1 *qian* of cooked Radix Aconiti Carmichaeli (*Shu Fu Zi*). In case of profuse sweating, add 1 *qian* of Radix Ephedrae Chinensis (*Ma Huang Geng*) and 1 handful of Fructus Levis Tritici (*Fu Xiao Mai*). In case of thirst, add 1 *qian* of Tuber Ophiopogonis Japonicae (*Mai Dong*) and 10 pieces of Fructus Schizandrae Chinensis (*Wu Wei Zi*). In case of constipation, add 1 *qian* of Herba Cistanchis (*Rou Cong Rong*) and a pinchful of Semen Cannabis Sativae (*Ma Ren*). In case of grain type food injury, add 1 *qian* of stir-fried Massa Medica Fermentata (*Shen Qu*) and 1 *qian* of stir-fried Fructus Germinatus Hordei Vulgaris (*Mai Ya*). In case of meat (type) food injury, add Fructus Crataegi (*Shan Zha*) and Fructus Seu Semen Amomi (*Sha Ren*), 5 *fen* each.

[Because (use of) Fructus Germinatus Hordei Vulgaris may run the risk of interrupting lactation, caution should be taken concerning its use. (The dosages of) Radix Astragali Seu Hedysari and Rhizoma Atractylodis Macrocephalae is (given as) 2 *qian* each in a variant edition. To stop sweating, it is proper to use stir-fried Fructus Levis Tritici.]

Wang Yan Wang Jian
Confused Speech, Confused Vision

Because qi and blood are vacuous, the *hun* and *po* or ethereal and corporeal souls have nothing on which to rely. Treatment depends on the presence or absence of lump pain as well as the degrees of acuteness. If lump pain is not yet relieved, one should first administer 2 or 3 *ji* of *Sheng Hua Tang*. When the pain is gone, change to *Jia Shen Sheng Hua Tang* or *Bu Zhong Yi*

Qi Tang combined with *An Shen Ding Zhi Wan* (Calm the Spirit & Stabilize Orientation Pill). If form and qi are both (still) insufficient long after delivery, it is imperative to greatly supplement the qi and blood and to calm the spirit and stabilize orientation. When these medicinals have built up sufficient strength (in the body), the disease will automatically be cured. Do not believe that this is obsession by an evil spirit. Spraying holy water, which can frighten (the patient), more often than not leads to incurability. (I have) treated quite a number of such cases where effect has refused to appear until well above 10 doses of this formula have been taken. This disease is (due to) vacuity, although it looks like an evil (repletion). To remove evils, first of all, supplement vacuity and regulate the qi. Then turn to the various signs. This is (the approach) that the ancients adopted in treating postpartum vacuity conditions, vacuity dyspnea at an advanced age, and ravings in weak persons. It merits careful consideration.

An Shen Sheng Hua Tang (Calm the Spirit Generating & Transforming Decoction) [Treats the conditions of postpartum raving and confused vision with lump pain which is not yet relieved. (In that case,) Radix Astragali Seu Hedysari (*Huang Qi*) and Rhizoma Atractylodis Macrocephalae (*Bai Zhu*) must not be used.]

Rhizoma Ligustici Wallichii (*Chuan Xiong*), 1 *qian*
Semen Biotae Orientalis (*Bai Zi Ren*), 1 *qian*
Radix Panacis Ginseng (*Ren Shen*), 1-2 *qian*
Radix Angelicae Sinensis (*Dang Gui*), 2-3 *qian*
Sclerotium Pararadicis Poriae Cocoris (*Fu Shen*), 2 *qian*
Semen Pruni Persicae (*Tao Ren*), 12 pieces
Rhizoma Carbonisata Zingiberis (*Hei Jiang*), 4 *fen*
Radix Praeparatus Glycyrrhizae (*Zhi Gan Cao*), 4 *fen*
Fructus Alpiniae Oxyphyllae (*Yi Zhi*), 8 *fen*, stir-fried
Pericarpium Citri Reticulatae (*Chen Pi*), 3 *fen*

Fructus Zizyphi Jujubae (*Zao*)

Decoct in water.

Zi Rong Yi Qi Fu Shen Tang (Enriching Construction, Boost the Qi, & Restore the Spirit Decoction) [If lump pain has already been relieved, take this formula and ravings and confused vision will be cured immediately.]

Radix Astragali Seu Hedysari (*Huang Qi*)
Rhizoma Atractylodis Macrocephalae (*Bai Zhu*)
Tuber Ophiopogonis Japonicae (*Mai Dong*)
Rhizoma Ligustici Wallichii (*Chuan Xiong*)
Semen Biotae Orientalis (*Bai Zi Ren*)
Sclerotium Pararadicis Poriae Cocoris (*Fu Shen*)
Fructus Alpiniae Oxyphyllae (*Yi Zhi*), each 1 *qian*
Pericarpium Citri Reticulatae (*Chen Pi*), 3 fen
Radix Panacis Ginseng (*Ren Shen*)
Radix Coquitus Rehmanniae (*Shu Di*), each 2 *qian*
Radix Praeparatus Glycyrrhizae (*Zhi Gan Cao*), 4 fen
Fructus Schizandrae Chinensis (*Wu Wei Zi*), 10 pieces
Semen Zizyphi Spinosae (*Zao Ren*), 10 pieces, 1 *qian*
Semen Nelumbinis Nuciferae (*Lian Zi*), 8 pieces
Arillus Euphoriae Longanae (*Yuan Rou*), 8 pieces
Fructus Zizyphi Jujubae (*Zao*)

Decoct in water.

Despite their separation into qi and blood, yin and yang (types), postpartum *xue beng*, blood desertion, dyspnea, qi desertion, spirit desertion, and raving all have in common beneath them dispersed essence and departed spirit. They appear later and are a little less acute than postpartum dizziness but are no less critical. Unless rich formulas are administered in quick succession, many deaths will occur. The allegation that qi repletion and phlegm fire (are responsible for these) is misleading. In case of blood lump pain shortly after delivery, administer *Jia Shen Sheng Hua Tang*. As supplementation is realized through moving (the blood), the danger of blood stagnation (and) blood dizziness is prevented. After lump pain is relieved, in order to treat blood desertion and to calm the blood so that it may return to the channels, it is proper to use *Sheng Ju Da Bu Tang* with a small amount of Rhizoma Coptidis Chinensis (*Huang Lian*) added as assistant to downbear fire. To treat qi desertion and to contain the qi so that it returns to the abyss, it is proper to use *Bu Zhong Yi Qi Tang* with a double amount of Radix Panacis Ginseng (*Ren Shen*) and a small amount of Radix Praeparatus Aconiti Carmichaeli (*Fu Zi*) added to assist Radix Panacis Ginseng. To clear heart fire and to calm the organ of the sovereign, it is appropriate to use *Zi Rong Yi Qi Fu Shen Tang* with a small amount of phlegm (eliminating) medicinals added as assistant.

Shang Shi
Food Injury

Shortly after delivery, one should abstain from fatty and refined foods and should stay away from rich flavors. An undisciplined diet inevitably injures the spleen and the stomach. Treatment should be to support the origin, warm and supplement the qi and blood, and fortify the spleen and the stomach. According to what substance is found to be the cause of the injury, certain abducting dispersion medicinals are added. To disperse cereal foods, add Massa Medica Fermentata (*Shen Qu*) and Fructus Germinatus Hordei Vulgaris (*Mai Ya*) to *Sheng Hua Tang*. Add Fructus Crataegi (*Shan Zha*) and Fructus Seu Semen Amomi (*Sha Ren*) to disperse meat food. In case of (injury due to overeating) cold foods, add Fructus Evodiae Rutaecarpae (*Wu Zhu*) and Cortex Cinnamomi (*Rou Gui*). In case of severe vacuity in the birthing woman, add Radix

Panacis Ginseng (*Ren Shen*) and Rhizoma Atractylodis Macrocephalae (*Bai Zhu*). If there are lumps in addition, simultaneous dispersion and supplementation can be used afterwards. Then an effect will show without fail. Physicians are not infrequently met who give no importance to postpartum weakness and know no better than to rapidly disperse what has brought about the injury, only to injure the *zhen* or true qi and make fullness and oppression all the more serious. How can caution not be taken?

Jia Wei Sheng Hua Tang (Added Flavors Generating & Transforming Decoction) [Taken to disperse food when blood clots are not yet eliminated]

Rhizoma Ligustici Wallichii (*Chuan Xiong*), 2 *qian*
Radix Angelicae Sinensis (*Dang Gui*), 5 *qian*
Rhizoma Carbonisata Zingiberis (*Hei Jiang*), 4 *fen*
Radix Praeparatus Glycyrrhizae (*Zhi Gan Cao*), 5 *fen*
Semen Pruni Persicae (*Tao Ren*), 10 pieces

Make certain of what has caused the injury and add and delete as above. Decoct in water.

Jian Pi Xiao Shi Sheng Hua Tang (Fortify the Spleen, Disperse Food Generating & Transforming Decoction) [Taken to disperse food after blood clots are eliminated.]

Rhizoma Ligustici Wallichii (*Chuan Xiong*), 1 *qian*
Radix Panacis Ginseng (*Ren Shen*)
Radix Angelicae Sinensis (*Dang Gui*), each 2 *qian*
Rhizoma Atractylodis Macrocephalae (*Bai Zhu*), 1.5 *qian*
Radix Praeparatus Glycyrrhizae (*Zhi Gan Cao*), 5 *fen*

In accordance with what is found to have caused the injury, add and subtract as above. If cold substances have been retained for a long time resulting in vacuity and weakness of the spleen and stomach, medicinals may fail to work. It is (then) necessary to use rubbing and pressing. It is still better to warm with stir-fried Massa Medica Fermentata (*Shen Qu*). In case of inability to take in (even) porridge for several days due misuse of abducting dispersion medicinals to treat food injury, it is always proper to administer this formula.

Fen Nu
Indignation (&) Anger

In case of postpartum anger (leading to) qi counterflow and inhibited chest and diaphragm with lump pain, it is proper to administer *Sheng Hua Tang* omitting Semen Pruni Persicae (*Tao Ren*). It is to be taken with 2 *fen* of rubbed Radix Saussureae Seu Vladimiriae (*Mu Xiang*) mixed in. Then the transformation of lumps and the dispersion of anger can be realized in a compatible way. If importance is given to the qi neglecting the postpartum condition and medicinals, such as Radix Saussureae Seu Vladimiriae, Radix Linderae Strychnifoliae (*Wu Yao*), Fructus Citri Seu Ponciri (*Zhi Qiao*), and Fructus Seu Semen Amomi (*Sha Ren*) are used exclusively, the original qi will, on the contrary, suffer injury, and fullness and oppression will mistakenly become more serious. If, additionally, a meal is eaten immediately after becoming angry, (resulting in) weak stomach and stagnation and oppression, one should make certain what substance has caused the injury and treat with the same method as above. Caution should be taken not to employ *Mu Xiang Bing Lang Wan* (Saussurea & Areca Pills)[5] or

5 These are composed of Radix Saussureae Seu Vladimiriae (*Mu Xiang*), Semen Arecae Catechu (*Bing Lang*), Pericarpium Viridis Citri Reticulatae (*Qing Pi*), Pericarpium Citri Reticulatae (*Chen Pi*), stir-fried Fructus Citri Seu Ponciri (*Zhi Qiao*), Rhizoma Coptidis Chinensis (*Huang Lian*), Rhizoma Sparganii (*San Leng*), Rhizoma Curcumae Zedoariae (*E Zhu*), 1 *liang each;* wine-fried Cortex

the *Liu Qi Yin Zi* (Flowing Qi Conductor),[6] since these will make vacuity and weakness worse.

Mu Xiang Sheng Hua Tang (Saussurea Generating & Transforming Decoction) [Treats postpartum suffering from anger with blood lumps already eliminated]

Rhizoma Ligustici Wallichii (*Chuan Xiong*), 2 *qian*
Radix Angelicae Sinensis (*Dang Gui*), 6 *qian*
Pericarpium Citri Reticulatae (*Chen Pi*), 3 *fen*
Rhizoma Carbonisata Zingiberis (*Hei Jiang*), 4 *fen*

Taken 2 *fen* of rubbed Radix Saussureae Seu Vladimiriae (*Mu Xiang*) mixed in. This formula is (a variant of *Sheng Hua Tang*) with Semen Pruni Persicae (*Tao Ren*) left out and Radix Saussurea Seu Vladimiriae and Pericarpium Citri Reticulatae added. In a preceding section there is (also) a variation with Rhizoma Desiccata Zingiberis (*Gan Jiang*) left out. Refer to it.

Phellodendri (*Huang Bai*), Radix Et Rhizoma Rhei (*Da Huang*), each 3 *liang;* and Rhizoma Cyperi Rotundi (*Xiang Fu*), Semen Pharbiditis (*Hei Chou*), each 4 *liang*. These are ground into a fine powder and made into pills 2 *qian* in weight.

6 This is composed of Pericarpium Arecae (*Da Fu Pi*), 1 *qian;* Pericarpium Citri Reticulatae (*Chen Pi*), Sclerotium Rubrum Poriae Cocoris (*Chi Fu Ling*), Radix Angelicae Sinensis (*Dang Gui*), Radix Albus Paeoniae Lactiflorae (*Bai Shao*), Rhizoma Ligustici Wallichii (*Chuan Xiong*), Radix Astragali Seu Hedysari (*Huang Qi*), Rhizoma Pinelliae Ternatae (*Ban Xia*), Fructus Immaturus Citri Seu Ponciri (*Zhi Shi*), Radix Glycyrrhizae (*Gan Cao*), Radix Ledebouriellae Sesloidis (*Fang Feng*), each 7.5 *fen;* Folium Perillae Frutescentis (*Su Ye*), Radix Linderae Strychnifoliae (*Wu Yao*), Pericarpium Viridis Citri Reticulatae (*Qing Pi*), Radix Platycodi Grandiflori (*Jie Geng*), each 1.5 *qian;* Radix Saussureae Seu Vladimiriae (*Mu Xiang*), 2.5 *fen;* 3 slices of Rhizoma Recens Zingiberis (*Jiang*); and 2 pieces of Fructus Zizyphi Jujubae (*Zao*).

Jian Pi Hua Shi San Qi Tang (Fortify the Spleen, Transform Food, & Dissipate the Qi Decoction) [Treats food injury due to angry qi without lump pain]

Rhizoma Atractylodis Macrocephalae (*Bai Zhu*), 2 *qian*
Radix Angelicae Sinensis (*Dang Gui*), 2 *qian*
Rhizoma Ligustici Wallichii (*Chuan Xiong*), 1 *qian*
Rhizoma Carbonisata Zingiberis (*Hei Jiang*), 4 *fen*
Radix Panacis Ginseng (*Ren Shen*), 2 *qian*
Pericarpium Citri Reticulatae (*Chen Pi*), 3 *qian*

In accordance with what is found to have caused the injury, add and subtract as above. Generally speaking, to treat the two conditions of postpartum qi counterflow provoked by indignation and anger and postpartum stagnation of food, a good physician should subordinate angry qi and dispersing food to the postpartum condition (in general) and always give priority to the supplementation of the qi and blood. When liver-regulation and qi-normalizing are used as assistants, the origin suffers no injury, while angry depression is dissipated. When spleen-fortification and abducting dispersion are used as assistants, stagnant food is moved and a desire for food (reappears). If one merely regulates the qi and disperses food, harm rather than good is done.

[In a variant edition, Pericarpium Citri Reticulatae is (given at) 3 *fen*, with 4 *fen* of Radix Glycyrrhizae (*Gan Cao*) also included.]

Lei Nue
Quasi-Malaria

Postpartum alternating fever and chills which attack daily at fixed intervals are like malaria in terms of (their) signs but should not be treated as malaria. It is because of qi and blood vacuity that fever and chills attack in an alternating way, and it is because of *yuan* or original qi vacuity that external evils invade. (Thus, the patient exhibits) rigid cold or extreme heat, is better by day but worse by night, or has late afternoon tidal fever. This is all perfectly similar to malaria. The proper treatment is to enrich construction and boost the qi to abate fever and chills. If sweating is present, it is imperative to stop it without delay. (This may) sometimes (be done) with the introduction of such medicinals as Radix Ephedrae Chinensis (*Ma Huang Geng*). Perspiration appearing merely on the head and failing to reach the feet is a critical condition of solitary yang with expiring yin. It is imperative to add such medicinals as Radix Coquitus Rehmanniae (*Di Huang*) and Radix Angelicae Sinensis (*Dang Gui*). Provided that the *yang ming* is without aversion to cold[7] but with headache and absence of sweating, simply administer *Sheng Hua Tang* with the addition of Radix Et Rhizoma Notopterygii (*Qiang Huo*), Radix Ledebouriellae Sesloidis (*Fang Feng*), root hairs of Rhizoma Coptidis Chinensis (*Huang Lian Xu*), and a number of Bulbus Allii Fistulosi (*Cong Bai*) for the purpose of dissipating. Formulas such as *Chai Hu Qing Gan Yin* (Bupleurum Clear the Liver Drink)[8] and agents like Radix Dichroae (*Chang Shan*) and Fructus Amomi Tsao-ko (*Cao Guo*) are all prohibited.

Zi Rong Yang Qi Fu Zheng Tang (Enrich Construction, Nurture the Qi, & Support the Righteous) [Treats postpartum fever and chills with sweating attacking regularly in the afternoon]

---

7 This refers to the *yang ming* pattern of cold injury which is subdivided into two: the channel pattern and the bowel pattern, each with different manifestations.

8 The ingredients of this formula are Radix Bupleuri (*Chai Hu*), Fructus Gardeniae Jasminoidis (*Zhi Zi*), Cortex Radicis Moutan (*Dan Pi*), Pericarpium Viridis Citri Reticulatae (*Qing Pi*), Radix Albus Paeoniae Lactiflorae (*Bai Shao*), Ramulus Perillae Frutescentis (*Su Geng*), and Ramus Uncariae Cum Uncis (*Gou Teng*).

Radix Panacis Ginseng (*Ren Shen*), 2 *qian*
Radix Praeparatus Astragali Seu Hedysari (*Zhi Huang Qi*)
Rhizoma Atractylodis Macrocephalae (*Bai Zhu*)
Rhizoma Ligustici Wallichii (*Chuan Xiong*)
Radix Coquitus Rehmanniae (*Shu Di*)
Tuber Ophiopogonis Japonicae (*Mai Dong*)
Radix Ephedrae Chinensis (*Ma Huang Geng*), each 1 *qian*
Radix Angelicae Sinensis (*Dang Gui*), 3 *qian*
Pericarpium Citri Reticulatae (*Chen Pi*), 4 *fen*
Radix Praeparatus Glycyrrhizae (*Zhi Gan Cao*), 5 *fen*
Fructus Zizyphi Jujubae (*Zao*)

Decoct in water.

Jia Jian Yang Wei Tang (Modified Nurture the Stomach Decoction) [Treats postpartum quasi-malaria with alternating fever and chills, headache, and absence of sweating]

Radix Praeparatus Glycyrrhizae (*Zhi Gan Cao*), 4 *fen*
Sclerotium Poriae Cocoris (*Bai Fu Ling*), 1 *qian*
Rhizoma Pinelliae Ternatae (*Ban Xia*), 8 *fen*, processed
Rhizoma Ligustici Wallichii (*Chuan Xiong*), 1 *qian*
Pericarpium Citri Reticulatae (*Chen Pi*), 4 *fen*
Radix Angelicae Sinensis (*Dang Gui*), 2 *qian*
Rhizoma Atractylodis (*Cang Zhu*), 1 *qian*
Herba Agastachis Seu Pogostemi (*Huo Xiang*), 4 *fen*
Radix Panacis Ginseng (*Ren Shen*), 1 *qian*
Fructus Zizyphi Jujubae (*Zao*), as conductor

Decoct and take.

In case of phlegm, add Succus Bambusae (*Zhu Li*), Succus Zingiberis (*Jiang Zhi*), Rhizoma Pinelliae Ternatae (*Ban Xia*), and Massa Medica Fermentata (*Shen Qu*). For a weak patient, also administer *He Che Wan* (Placenta Pills).[9] In case of enduring malaria which will not heal, simultaneously administer *Shen Zhu Gao* (Ginseng & Atractylodes Paste) to aid the strength of the decoction.

Shen Zhu Gao (Ginseng & Atractylodes Paste)

Soak 1 *jin* of Rhizoma Atractylodis Macrocephalae (*Bai Zhu*) in rice water for 1 night, powder, and bake in a pot. Boil this with 1 *liang* of Radix Panacis Ginseng (*Ren Shen*) in 6 bowls of water down to 2 bowls. The dregs are to be boiled twice more so that (one) has 6 bowlfuls of decoction altogether. Put these all together and boil down to 1 bowlful. Dissolve half a cup of this paste in thin rice porridge and take it on an empty stomach.

Lei Shang Han Er Yang Zheng Quasi-Cold Injury Conditions of the Two Yang

(If,) within seven days after delivery, (a woman exhibits) fever, headache, and aversion to cold, this cannot be categorically classified as a *tai yang* pattern of *shang han* or cold injury. Nor can fever, headache, and lateral costal pain be categorically classified as a *shao yang* pattern of *shang han*. These two patterns are both (typically) subsumed under external invasion, but (postpartum) they are caused by dual vacuity of qi and blood and disharmony between yin and yang. The physician should not overlook the postpartum heat category and

---

9 These are composed of Placenta Hominis (*He Che*), Sclerotium Poriae Cocoris (*Fu Ling*), Radix Polygalae Tenuifoliae (*Yuan Zhi*), 1 *liang* each; Radix Panacis Ginseng (*Ren Shen*), 5 *qian*; and Radix Salviae Miltorrhizae (*Dan Shen*), 7 *qian*. Prepare as pills 3 *qian* in weight.

prescribe *Ma Huang Tang* (Ephedra Decoction) in treating a quasi-*tai yang* pattern or *Chai Hu Tang* (Bupleurum Decoction) in treating a quasi-*shao yang* pattern. What's more, if a birth mother who has sustained blood desertion receives sudorific (treatment), the emptying (of what is already) empty may bring unpredictable (and) disastrous consequences. (Zhang) Zhong-jing said, "Patients with blood collapse cannot be treated by diaphoresis." (Zhu) Dan-xi said, "Exterior effusion should never be applied to postpartum cases for any reason." These two masters do not actually mean that there is no (possibility of) postpartum complications (due to) cold damage or that *Ma Huang Tang* and *Chai Hu Tang* are not appropriate for their indicated patterns. However, they cherished a fear that beginners in later generations, taking a one-sided view and overlooking the postpartum condition, would stick to proven formulas and apply exterior effusion. It should be understood that, in case of true invasion of wind or cold, *Sheng Hua Tang* does have Rhizoma Ligustici Wallichii (*Chuan Xiong*) and Rhizoma Zingiberis (*Jiang*) to dissipate these.

Jia Wei Sheng Hua Tang (Added Flavors Generating & Transforming Decoction) [Treats fever and headache within three days after delivery]

Rhizoma Ligustici Wallichii (*Chuan Xiong*)
Radix Ledebouriellae Sesloidis (*Fang Feng*), each 1 *qian*
Radix Angelicae Sinensis (*Dang Gui*), 3 *qian*
Radix Praeparatus Glycyrrhizae (*Zhi Gan Cao*), 4 *fen*
Semen Pruni Persicae (*Tao Ren*), 10 pieces
Radix Et Rhizoma Notopterygii (*Qiang Huo*), 4 *fen*

[In a variant edition, there is no Semen Pruni Persicae. There is Rhizoma Carbonisata Zingiberis (*Hei Jiang*), 4 *fen*.

A word of clarification on the deletion of Semen Pruni Persicae from that edition: Its deletion can be questioned only after the presence or absence of lump pain are ascertained. If headache and body heat or generalized fever persist after 2 *jis* are taken, add 8 fen of Radix Angelicae (*Bai Zhi*) and 4 fen of Herba Cum Radice Asari Sieboldi (*Xi Xin*). If fever refuses to abate and headache remains the same as before, add 5 stalks of Allium Fistulosum (*Cong*) with roots and 3 *qian* of Radix Panacis Ginseng (*Ren Shen*). Since not yet dispersed, postpartum vanquished blood can also be a cause of alternating fever and chills. How is this identified? The answer is that intermittent, pricking pain indicates vanquished blood; while merely alternating fever and chills without complications indicates disharmony between yin and yang. In case of pricking pain, use Radix Angelicae Sinensis (*Dang Gui*) which is a blood-harmonizing medicinal. If the pricking pain is due to accumulated blood, it is proper to use medicinals such as Flos Carthami Tinctorii (*Hong Hua*), Semen Pruni Persicae (*Tao Ren*), and Apex Radicis Angelicae Sinensis (*Gui Wei*).]

Lei Shang Han San Yin Zheng
Quasi-Cold Injury Conditions of the Three Yin

Tidal fever with sweating and constipation cannot be categorically classified as a *yang ming* condition. Dry mouth and throat with thirst cannot be categorically classified as a *shao yin* condition. Abdominal fullness with desiccated fluids and solid stools cannot be categorically classified as a *tai yin* condition. Nor can sweating, delirious raving, and constipation be categorically classified as a condition of dry stools in the stomach and intestines indicating precipitation or descension. These several conditions are, in most cases, caused by injury of the spleen by taxation and fatigue, retarded transportation and transformation, wasted qi and blood, and dried up intestines and bowels. These are vacuity conditions which are similar to replete conditions and which require supplementation. Physicians should not adhere to a one-sided view and overlook the postpartum condition, nor thereby indiscreetly suggest the three *Cheng Qi Tang* (Support the Qi Decoctions)[10] to treat these three quasi-yin conditions. There are indeed very few cases of young, strong women who have luckily come to no harm after being unwarrantedly treated with precipitation. And, after giving birth, most weak and feeble (patients) after being so treated are reduced to incurability. It is not infrequently seen that unwarranted precipitation leads, on the contrary, to inflation. Inappropriate abduction results, on the contrary, in binding. There are also (cases where constipation due to) shortage of blood have been abruptly turned to unstoppable diarrhea by precipitation which has lasted for several days. This is dangerous! It is stated in the *Fu Ren Liang Fang (Fine Formulas for Women)* [11]:

> (If) postpartum constipation with much food intake, based on the number of days it has lasted, is treated with medicinals to relax the bowels, disastrous consequences will presently befall.

Not until the abdomen is felt full and distended, with a desire but inability to move (the bowels), when binding has occurred in the rectum, is it proper to moisten (the intestine) with pig

10 These are *Da Cheng Qi Tang* (Major Support the Qi Decoction), *Xiao Cheng Qi Tang* (Minor Support the Qi Decoction), and *Tiao Wei Cheng Qi Tang* (Balance the Stomach, Support the Qi Decoction).

11 This is a famous compendium of gynecological formulae compiled by Chen Zi-ming and published in 1237 CE. It is also sometimes referred to as *Fu Ren Liang Fang Da Quan* or *The Great Compendium of Fine Formulas for Women*. It was the first systematic work specializing in *fu ke* or gynecology in Chinese medicine.

bile. If food is taken as usual and there is no anomaly in relation to the abdomen, though constipation has lasted long, nothing but supplementing medicinals should be used. If bitter, cold medicinals are administered to dredge, central qi will be, on the contrary, injured. Though open, the bowels may not stop. Or glomus and fullness might develop. This is erroneous!

Yang Zheng Tong You Tang (Nurture the Righteous, Free the Dark Decoction) [Treats postpartum constipation in the three quasi-cold injury yin conditions]

Rhizoma Ligustici Wallichii (*Chuan Xiong*), 2.5 *qian*
Radix Angelicae Sinensis (*Dang Gui*), 6 *qian*
Radix Praeparatus Glycyrrhizae (*Zhi Gan Cao*), 5 *fen*
Semen Pruni Persicae (*Tao Ren*), 15 pieces
Semen Cannabis Sativae (*Ma Ren*), 2 *qian*, stir-fried
Herba Cistanchis (*Rou Cong Rong*), washed with wine, scaled, 1 *qian*

In case of copious sweating and solid stools, add 1 *qian* of Radix Astragali Seu Hedysari (*Huang Qi*), 1 *qian* of Radix Ephedrae Chinensis (*Ma Huang Geng*), and 2 *qian* of Radix Panacis Ginseng (*Ren Shen*). In case of dry mouth and thirst, add Radix Panacis Ginseng and Tuber Ophiopogonis Japonicae (*Mai Dong*), each 1 *qian*. In case of over-full abdomen and solid stools, add 1 *qian* of Tuber Ophiopogonis Japonicae, 6 fen of Fructus Citri Seu Ponciri (*Zhi Qiao*), 2 *qian* of Radix Panacis Ginseng, and 1 *qian* of Herba Cistanchis (*Rou Cong Rong*). In case of sweating, delirious raving, and solid stools which are due to qi and blood vacuity and exhaustion and to essence spirit failing to keep to (their abode), it is proper to nurture the *ying* and calm the spirit by adding Sclerotium Pararadicis Poriae Cocoris (*Fu Shen*), Radix Polygalae Tenuifoliae (*Yuan Zhi*), Herba Cistanchis, 1 *qian* each, Radix Panacis Ginseng and

Rhizoma Atractylodis Macrocephalae (*Ba Zhu*), 2 *qian* each, Radix Astragali Seu Hedysari (*Huang Qi*) and Radix Angelicae (*Bai Zhi*), 1 *qian* each, and 1 *qian* of Semen Biotae Orientalis (*Bai Zi Ren*).

The above several conditions of dry, bound stools hardly show improvement before one consumes as much as one *jin* of Radix Angelicae Sinensis and Radix Panacis Ginseng. Generally speaking, even though postpartum vacuity with cold injury and food injury exhibits external signs of headache and fever or lateral costal and lumbar pain, (typically signs of) the external invasion indicative of diaphoresis, priority should, nevertheless, be given to the postpartum condition. (In this case,) diaphoresis is prohibited due to blood collapse. The only appropriate choice is *Sheng Hua Tang* which can be modified according to the specific conditions. It will unfailingly achieve regulation and rectification. This is true of constipation. Likewise, because priority is given to the postpartum condition, precipitation is prohibited due to blood collapse. It is proper to nurture the righteous and assist blood to free stagnation. This is the safe (way).

Additionally, ***Run Chang Zhou*** (Moisten the Intestines Gruel) [Treats enduring postpartum fecal stoppage]

Take 1 *shen* of Semen Sesami Indicae (*Zhi Ma*), grind coarsely, and mix with 2 *he* of rice. Boil into gruel and take. When the intestines are moistened, (stoppage) is freed.

Lei Zhong Feng
Quasi-Windstroke

With delivery, the qi and blood become abruptly vacuous, and the hundreds of bones are short of blood to moisten and nourish them. Quasi-windstroke, epileptic tetany with suddenly clenched jaws and teeth, hypertonicity of the sinews of the hands and feet, and the like should be treated as the branch even if vacuity fire is flaming upward with phlegm. One should not adhere to a one-sided view and prescribe wind-treating and phlegm-dispersing formulas, thus inflicting double vacuity on the birthing woman. The appropriate treatment method is, first of all, to administer *Sheng Hua Tang* to generate and make effulgent new blood. In critical cases, after 3 *ji* are taken, it is necessary to change to *Jia Shen* (Added Ginseng formula) in order to boost qi to salvage deserted blood. In case of phlegm fire, add a small amount of Exocarpium Citri Rubri (*Ju Hong*), stir-fried Radix Scutellariae Baicalensis (*Huang Qin*), or the like. Succus Bambusae (*Zhu Li*) or Succus Zingiberis (*Jiang Zhi*) can be added also, but Rhizoma Coptidis Chinensis (*Huang Lian*) and Cortex Phellodendri (*Huang Bai*) should not be used together. Be cautious!

Zi Rong Huo Luo Tang (Enrich Construction, Activate the Connecting Vessels Decoction) [Treats the postpartum quasi-wind condition of shortage of blood, clenched jaws, rigidity of the neck, and hypertonicity of the sinews]

Rhizoma Ligustici Wallichii (*Chuan Xiong*), 1.5 *qian*
Radix Angelicae Sinensis (*Dang Gui*)
Radix Coquitus Rehmanniae (*Shu Di*)
Radix Panacis Ginseng (*Ren Shen*), each 2 *qian*
Radix Astragali Seu Hedysari (*Huang Qi*)
Sclerotium Pararadicis Poriae Cocoris (*Fu Shen*)
Rhizoma Gastrodiae Elatae (*Tian Ma*), each 1 *qian*
Radix Praeparatus Glycyrrhizae (*Zhi Gan Cao*)
Pericarpium Citri Reticulatae (*Chen Pi*)
Herba Seu Flos Schizonepetae Tenuifoliae (*Jing Jie Sui*)
Radix Ledebouriellae Sesloidis (*Fang Feng*)
Radix Et Rhizoma Notopterygii (*Qiang Huo*), each 4 *fen*

Rhizoma Coptidis Chinensis (*Huang Lian*), 8 *fen*, stir-fried with ginger juice

In case of phlegm, add Succus Bambusae (*Zhu Li*), Succus Zingiberis (*Jiang Zhi*), and Rhizoma Pinelliae Ternatae (*Ban Xia*). In case of thirst, add Tuber Ophiopogonis Japonicae (*Mai Dong*) and Radix Puerariae Lobatae (*Ge Geng*). In case of food (injury), add Fructus Crataegi (*Shan Zha*) and Fructus Seu Semen Amomi (*Sha Ren*) to disperse meat food or Massa Medica Fermentata (*Shen Qu*) and Fructus Germinatus Hordei Vulgaris (*Mai Ya*) to disperse grain food. In case of fecal stoppage, add 1.5 *qian* of Herba Cistanchis (*Rou Cong Rong*). In case of copious sweating, add 1 *qian* of Radix Ephedrae Chinensis (*Ma Huang Geng*). In case of fright palpitations, add 1 *qian* of Semen Zizyphi Spinosae (*Zao Ren*).

Tian Ma Wan (Gastrodia Pills) [Treats postpartum wind stroke with abstraction, difficult speech, and inhibition of the four limbs.]

Rhizoma Gastrodiae Elatae (*Tian Ma*), 1 *qian*
Radix Ledebouriellae Sesloidis (*Fang Feng*), 1 *qian*
Rhizoma Ligustici Wallichii (*Chuan Xiong*), 7 *fen*
Radix Et Rhizoma Notopterygii (*Qiang Huo*), 7 *fen*
Radix Panacis Ginseng (*Ren Shen*)
Radix Polygalae Tenuifoliae (*Yuan Zhi*)
Semen Biotae Orientalis (*Bai Zi Ren*)
Radix Dioscoreae Oppositae (*Shan Yao*)
Tuber Ophiopogonis Japonicae (*Mai Dong*), each 1 *qian*
Semen Zizyphi Spinosae (*Zao Ren*), 1 *liang*
Herba Cum Radice Asari Sieboldi (*Xi Xin*), 1 *qian*
Massa Medica Fermentata Cum Rhizomatis Arisaematis (*Nan Xing Qu*), 8 *fen*
Rhizoma Acori Graminei (*Shi Chang Pu*), 1 *qian*

Grind into a fine powder, mix with heated honey, and make into pills coated with Cinnabaris (*Zhu Sha*). Take 60-70 pills with boiled water (as a *ji*).

[In a variant edition, Semen Zizyphi Spinosae is 1 *qian* and Herba Cum Radice Asari Sieboldi is 4 *qian*.]

Lei Jing
Quasi-Tetany

(If) postpartum there is profuse sweating followed, in addition, by tetany or convulsions manifested by rigidity of the nape (of the neck) and arched back (*i.e.*, opisthotonos) with breathing as if (on the point of) expiration, it is necessary to immediately administer *Jia Jian Sheng Hua Tang* (Modified Generating & Transforming Decoction).

Jia Jian Sheng Hua Tang (Modified Generating & Transforming Decoction) [Specifically treats sweating accompanied by tetany]

Rhizoma Ligustici Wallichii (*Chuan Xiong*)
Herba Ephedrae Chinensis (*Ma Huang Geng*), each 1 *qian*
Radix Angelicae Sinensis (*Dang Gui*), 4 *qian*
Ramulus Cinnamomi (*Gui Zhi*), 5 *fen*
Radix Panacis Ginseng (*Ren Shen*), 1 *qian*
Radix Praeparatus Glycyrrhizae (*Zhi Gan Cao*), 5 *fen*
Radix Et Rhizoma Notopterygii (*Qiang Huo*), 5 *fen*
Rhizoma Gastrodiae Elatae (*Tian Ma*), 8 *fen*
Radix Praeparatus Aconiti Carmichaeli (*Fu Zi*), 1 slice
Cornu Antelopis Saigae Tartaricae (*Ling Yang Jiao*), 8 *fen*

In case of quasi-tetanic windstroke without sweating, use 3 *qian* of Rhizoma Ligustici Wallichii (*Chuan Xiong*) and 1 *liang* of wine-washed Radix Anglicae Sinensis (*Dang Gui*) in addition to Semen Zizyphi Spinosae (*Zao Ren*) and Radix Ledebouriellae Sesloidis (*Fang Feng*), both in indefinite amounts.

[A variant edition has 1 slice of Rhizoma Recens Zingiberis (*Jiang*) and 1 piece Fructus Zizyphi Jujubae (*Zao*) in addition.]

Chu Han
Sweating

Sweating in the course of labor is usually caused by taxation injury of the spleen, fright injury of the heart, or worry injury of the liver. Most birthing women have (all) three (of these) simultaneously and (therefore) the perspiration. It is not permissible at that time to administer perspiration-constraining formulas. When the spirit becomes tranquil, perspiration will stop by itself. (In case of sweating with) blood clots causing pain, Radix Astragali Seu Hedysari (*Huang Qi*) or Rhizoma Atractylodis Macrocephalae (*Bai Zhu*) may not be used for the time being. It is appropriate to administer 2-3 *ji* of *Sheng Hua Tang* to relieve lump pain and then to administer *Jia Shen Sheng Hua Tang* (Added Ginseng Generating & Transforming Decoction) to stop vacuity sweating. If severe fatigue follows delivery, incessant sweating with form and complexion desertion are a desertion sweating with collapsed yang. Sweating can lead to collapse of yang. When yang collapses, yin follows. Therefore, this particular condition should be taken into account. Immediately pour down (the throat of the patient) *Jia Shen Sheng Hua Tang* with a double amount of Radix Panacis Ginseng (*Ren Shen*) to rescue the crisis without regard to clot or lump pain. In case of copious sweating in the birthing woman during labor, it is imperative to fortify the spleen to constrain the essence of water/fluids and to boost the *ying* and *wei*, thus urging the blood to return to the source. Therefore, the blood may irrigate the four limbs and be kept from flowing in a reckless way. In terms of miscellaneous conditions, sweating is classified as (either) *zi han* or spontaneous sweating or *dao han,* thief or night sweating. *Dang Gui Liu Huang Tang* (*Dang Gui* Six Yellows Decoction)[12], however, is not an appropriate formula to treat postpartum night sweating. The two formulas which are appropriate to administer are *Jia Shen Sheng Hua Tang* and *Jia Wei Bu Zhong Yi Qi (Tang)* (Added Flavors Supplement the Center, Boost the Qi Decoction). If sweating becomes (even) more profuse and unstoppable after Radix Panacis Ginseng and Radix Astragali Seu Hedysari are taken or sweat appears merely on the head but is absent from the lumbar region down to the feet, this must be a difficult case. If sweat pours so (quickly) so that the hand does not have enough time to wipe it off, the case is incurable. Postpartum sweating, dyspnea, and the like are extreme vacuity conditions. If incompatible with supplementation, the case is incurable.

Ma Huang Geng Tang (Ephedra Decoction) [Treats incessant postpartum vacuity sweating]

Radix Panacis Ginseng (*Ren Shen*), 2 *qian*
Radix Angelicae Sinensis (*Dang Gui*), 2 *qian*
Radix Praeparatus Astragali Seu Hedysari (*Zhi Huang Qi*), 1.5 *qian*
Rhizoma Atractylodis Macrocephalae (*Bai Zhu*), 1 *qian*, stir-fried
Ramulus Cinnamomi (*Gui Zhi*), 5 *fen*
Radix Ephedrae Chinensis (*Ma Huang Geng*), 1 *qian*
Radix Glycyrrhizae (*Fen Cao*), 5 *fen*, de-barked (&) stir-fried
Concha Ostreae (*Mu Li*), ground, a tiny amount
Fructus Levis Tritici (*Fu Xiao Mai*), a big handful

---

12 This formula is composed of Radix Coquitus Rehmanniae (*Shu Di*), Radix Rehmanniae (*Sheng Di*), Radix Scutellariae Baicalensis (*Huang Qin*), Cortex Phellodendri (*Huang Bai*), Rhizoma Coptidis Chinensis (*Huang Lian*), Radix Astragalus Seu Hedysari (*Huang Qi*), and Radix Angelicae Sinensis (*Dang Gui*).

In case of vacuity desertion with copious sweating and cold hands and feet, add 4 *fen* of Rhizoma Carbonisata Zingiberis (*Hei Jiang*) and 1 slice of Radix Praeparatus Aconiti Carmichaeli (*Fu Zi*). In case of thirst, add 1 *qian* of Tuber Ophiopogonis Japonicae (*Mai Dong*) and 10 pieces of Fructus Schizandrae Chinensis (*Wu Wei*). For a fat, white woman with copious postpartum sweating, add 1 cup of Succus Bambusae (*Zhu Li*) and a small spoonful of Succus Zingiberis (*Jiang Zhi*) to clear phlegm fire. In case of aversion to wind and cold, add Radix Ledebouriellae Sesloidis (*Fang Feng*) and Ramulus Cinnamomi (*Gui Zhi*), each 5 *fen*. In case of retention of blood clots, add 3 *qian* of Radix Coquitus Rehmanniae (*Shu Di*) and take ***Ba Wei Di Huang Wan*** (Eight Flavors Rehmanniae Pills) at night.

Fructus Corni Officinalis (*Shan Zhu Yu*)
Radix Dioscoreae Oppositae (*Shan Yao*)
Cortex Radicis Moutan (*Dan Pi*)
Sclerotium Poriae Cocoris (*Yun Ling*), each 8 *qian*
Rhizoma Alismatis (*Ze Xie*), 5 *qian*
Radix Coquitus Rehmanniae (*Shu Di*), 8 *qian*
Fructus Schizandra Chinensis (*Wu Wei Zi*), 5 *qian*
Radix Praeparatus Astragali Seu Hedysari (*Zhi Huang Qi*), 1 *liang*

Mix with heated honey and make into pills. There are cases of sweating which, arising whenever yang adds to yin, results in tugging and slackening if encountered by wind. These are particularly difficult to treat. For that reason, (a person) with copious sweating should carefully keep out of wind and cold. Profuse sweating with urination not free is the result of *jin ye* or fluid collapse and, (therefore,) water disinhibiting medicinals are prohibited.

Dao Han
Thief (*i.e.*, Night) Sweating

After delivery, perspiration appearing during sleep but disappearing on awakening is called *dao han* or thief sweating since it behaves like a thief peeping in at a sleeping person. There is no comparison between it and the perspiration that comes spontaneously. The *Za Zheng Lun (The Treatise on Miscellaneous Conditions)*[13] says, "Spontaneous sweating (is due to) yang depletion; while thief sweating (is due to) yin vacuity." However, again *Dang Gui Liu Huang Tang* (*Dang Gui* Six Yellows Decoction) is not the appropriate formula to treat postpartum thief or night sweating. Only that which (can) regulate the qi and blood in addition (to stopping sweating) is appropriate.

Zhi Han San (Stop Sweating Powder) [Treats postpartum thief sweating]

Radix Panacis Ginseng (*Ren Shen*), 2 *qian*
Radix Angelicae Sinensis (*Dang Gui*), 2 *qian*
Radix Coquitus Rehmanniae (*Shu Di*), 1.5 *qian*
Radix Ephedrae Chinensis (*Ma Huang Geng*), 5 *fen*
Rhizoma Coptidis Chinensis (*Huang Lian*), 5 *fen*, stir-fried with wine
Fructus Levis Tritici (*Fu Xiao Mai*), 1 big handful
Fructus Zizyphi Jujubae (*Da Zao*) 1 piece

Another Formula:

---

13 This is part of Zhang Jing-yue's complete writings, called in Chinese, *Jing Yue Quan Shu*. It is 29 volumes or books in length. Zhang Jing-yue is also known as Zhang Jie-bin and lived from 1563-1640 CE.

Concha Ostreae (*Mu Li*), calcined to fine powder, 5 *fen*
Pulvis Fructi Tritici (*Xiao Mai Mian*), fried yellow, powdered fine

[A variant edition (gives) Concha Ostreae and Pulvis Fructi Tritici, each 5 five *fen*, to be taken on an empty stomach.]

Kou Ke Jian Xiao Bian Bu Li
Thirsty Mouth (with) Simultaneous Inhibited Urination

Postpartum vexation, agitation, dry throat, and thirst with inhibited urination are the result of loss of blood and copious sweating. The treatment should be to assist the spleen, boost the lungs, and lift the qi and blood. Thus yang will ascend, while yin will descend. Water enters the channels to transform into blood and fluids; while grains enter the stomach so that qi grows and the pulse moves. As a result, fluids are naturally generated and urination is balanced and disinhibited. If Radix Scutellariae Baicalensis (*Huang Qin*), Rhizoma Coptis Chinensis (*Huang Lian*), Fructus Gardeniae Jasminoidis (*Zhi Zi*), or Cortex Phellodendri (*Huang Bai*) are used to downbear (fire) on the assumption that thirst is ascribed to fire, or, if one uses *Wu Ling San* to free (the flow) on the assumption that inhibited urination is ascribed to stagnated water, these are erroneous treatments. It is imperative to warm and boost in view of fatigue and detriment and to moisten and move in view of retention and stagnation. Then success is not far off.

Sheng Jin Zhi Ke Yi Shui Yin (Generate Fluids, Quench Thirst, & Boost Water Drink)

Radix Panacis Ginseng (*Ren Shen*)
Tuber Ophiopogonis Japonicae (*Mai Dong*)

Radix Angelicae Sinensis (*Dang Gui*)
Radix Rehmanniae (*Sheng Di*), each 3 *qian*
Radix Astragali Seu Hedysari (*Huang Qi*), 1 *qian*
Radix Puerariae Lobatae (*Ge Geng*), 1 *qian*
Rhizoma Cimicifugae (*Sheng Ma*)
Radix Praeparatus Glycyrrhizae (*Zhi Gan Cao*), each 4 *fen*
Sclerotium Poriae Cocoris (*Fu Ling*), 8 *fen*
Fructus Schizandrae Chinensis (*Wu Wei Zi*), 15 seeds

In case of profuse sweating, add 1 *qian* of Radix Ephedrae Chinensis (*Ma Huang Geng*) and 1 large handful of Fructus Levis Tritici (*Fu Xiao Mai*). In case of dry stools, add 1.5 *qian* of Herba Cistanchis (*Rou Cong Rong*). In case of severe thirst, add *Sheng Mai San* (Generate the Pulse Powder). Do not doubt this and, therefore, not use it.

Wei Niao
Enuresis

(This is due to) extreme qi vacuity and blood failing to retain (water). It is appropriate (to use) *Ba Zhen Tang* (Eight Pearls Decoction) plus Rhizoma Cimicifugae (*Sheng Ma*) and Radix Bupleuri (*Chai Hu*). In serious cases, add 1 slice of cooked Radix Praeparatus Aconiti Carmichaeli (*Fu Zi*).

Book 4

Chan Hou
Birthing & Afterwards (Continued)

Chan Hou
Birthing & Afterwards (Continued)

Wu Po Niao Bao
Mistaken Damage of the Urinary Bladder

In case of an inadvertently damaged bladder due to problems during delivery and an ill-practiced midwife, use Radix Panacis Ginseng (*Ren Shen*) and Radix Astragali Seu Hedysari (*Huang Qi*) as the rulers, Radix Angelicae Sinensis (*Dang Gui*) and Rhizoma Ligustici Wallichii (*Chuan Xiong*) as the ministers, and Semen Pruni Persicae (*Tao Ren*), Pericarpium Citri Reticulatae (*Chen Pi*), and Sclerotium Poriae Cocoris (*Fu Ling*) as the assistants. Decoct these medicinals with a pig or sheep's urinary bladder. 100 *ji* ensure safety. Another formula says to boil 1 *chi* of raw yellow silk cloth, powdered white Cortex Radicis Moutan (*Mu Dan Pi*), and powdered Rhizoma Bletillae Striatae (*Bai Ji*), each 2 *qian*, together in 2 bowls of water till the cloth is dissolved and becomes maltlike. After taking the decoction, it is proper to lie down quietly without speaking. (This formula) is called *Bu Pao Yin* (Mend the Bladder Drink) and is miraculously effective.

Huan Lin
Contraction of Strangury

(This is) due to postpartum vacuity and weakness with heat settling in the bladder. Internal vacuity makes urination frequent, while heat makes urination dribbling, inhibited, and painful. (This is) called *lin* or strangury.

Mao Geng Tang (Imperata Decoction) [Treats postpartum strangury, either cold or hot]

Gypsum (*Shi Gao*), 1 *liang*
Rhizoma Imperatae Cylindricae (*Bai Mao Geng*), 1 *liang*
Herba Dianthi (*Qu Mai*)
Sclerotium Poriae Cocoris (*Bai Fu Ling*), each 5 *qian*
Semen Abutiloni Seu Malvae (*Kui Zi*)
Radix Panacis Ginseng (*Ren Shen*)
Gummum Pruni Persicae (*Tao Jiao*)
Talcum (*Hua Shi*), each 1 *qian*
Caput Pseudosciaenae Crocerae (*Shi Shou Yu Tou*), 4 pieces

Decoct with Medulla Junci Effusi (*Deng Xin*) with powdered teeth mixed (in at the end) and take on an empty stomach.

[There is a note in a variant edition: If the condition is due to internal vacuity, use 1 *liang* of Gypsum. This treatment method is impossible. Do not adhere blindly to the old formulas and thus harm the patient. In another variant edition, Gypsum is (given at) 1 *qian* and there is no Talcum. Still another variant edition prescribes equal amounts (of these).]

Another formula [Treats postpartum dribbling urination with pain and blood in the urine]

Rhizoma Imperatae Cylindricae (*Bai Mao Geng*)

Herba Dianthi (*Qu Mai*)
Semen Abutilonis Seu Malvae (*Kui Zi*)
Semen Plantaginis (*Che Qian Zi*)
Medulla Tetrapanacis Papyriferi (*Tong Cao*), no definite amounts for the above
Teeth of carp, 100 pieces

Decoct in water and take. Also take powdered teeth.

[Note that the powdered teeth in both formulae are thought to be the carp's teeth.]

Bian Shu
Frequent Urination

(This is) due to chilly qi existing originally within the (space of the) bladder. Because delivery sets this in motion, this chilly qi enters the (tissue of the) bladder. Take 2 *liang* of powdered Hallyositum Rubrum (*Chi Shi Zhi*) on an empty stomach.

Another formula treats frequent urination and enuresis. Use 28 pieces of Fructus Alpiniae Oxyphyllae (*Yi Zhi Ren*) and powder. Take 2 *qian* (of this powder) with thin rice porridge.

Additionally, ***Sang Piao San*** (Ootheca Mantidis Powder)

Ootheca Mantidis (*Sang Piao Xiao*), 30 pieces
Radix Panacis Ginseng (*Ren Shen*)
Radix Astragali Seu Hedysari (*Huang Qi*)
Cornu Cervi Parvum (*Lu Rong*)
Concha Ostreae (*Mu Li*)
Hallyositum Rubrum (*Chi Shi Zhi*), each 3 *qian*

Powder. Take 2 *qian* on an empty stomach with thin rice porridge.

Xie
Diarrhea

Unlike in miscellaneous conditions, postpartum diarrhea is not classified into food diarrhea, damp diarrhea, and downpouring of water and grains diarrhea. Roughly speaking, it is (either due to) qi vacuity, food accumulation, or dampness. Vacuity requires supplementation; food accumulation requires dispersion; and dampness requires drying. However, when the lochia has not yet cleared up, it is hardly possible to apply drying right away. It is, (therefore,) necessary to first administer 2-3 doses of *Sheng Hua Tang* to transform the stale and generate the new, with Sclerotium Poriae Cocoris (*Fu Ling*) added to disinhibit the water passageways. After blood has been generated, (one should) supplement the qi to disperse food and dry dampness, (thus) diverting and disinhibiting the water passageways. This prevents the trouble of stagnating the inhibited and emptying (what is already) empty. Only after 10 days after delivery can diarrhea be regarded as a *za zheng* or miscellaneous disease. Nevertheless, (even its) treatment must still especially be designed in terms of vacuity and repletion. Watery stools with pain, abdominal rumbling, and inability to transform (even) thin rice porridge should be treated as cold diarrhea. Reddish yellow, watery stools with pain around the anus should be treated as hot diarrhea. (If the stools) smell like rotten eggs due to injury of the spleen by overeating, this should be treated as food accumulation. In addition, cases with persisting empty spleen qi, low food intake, rumbling on ingestion with relief experienced only after having instantly voided what was eaten should be treated as *xu han* or empty cold diarrhea. The treatment methods are to warm in case of cold, to clear in case of heat, and to disinhibit diversion and fortify the spleen in case of injured spleen and food accumulation. (If one) combines dispersing with the supplementation of vacuity, and well designs a balancing treatment, there will be no failure. Postpartum vacuity diarrhea with lethargy, somnolence, and loss of consciousness is a critical condition of extreme weakness and form desertion. To rescue life, it is necessary to use 2 *qian* of Radix Panacis Ginseng (*Ren Shen*), 2 qian each of Rhizoma Atractylodis Macrocephalae (*Bai Zhu*) and Sclerotium Poriae Cocoris (*Fu Ling*), and 1 *qian* of Radix Praeparatus Aconiti Carmichaeli (*Fu Zi*). If the pulse is floating and wiry and when pressed does not beat (forcefully), this is cold in the center. This is (a case of) yin collapsing first with yang already on the verge of departure. It is proper to greatly and immediately supplement the qi and blood and to add Radix Praeparatus Aconiti Carmichaeli and Rhizoma Carbonisata Zingiberis (*Hei Jiang*) to recover yang. It does not allow for a thread of negligence.

Jia Jian Sheng Hua Tang (Modified Generating & Transforming Decoction) [Treats postpartum diarrhea with clots not yet eliminated]

Rhizoma Ligustici Wallichii (*Chuan Xiong*), 2 *qian*
Sclerotium Poriae Cocoris (*Fu Ling*), 2 *qian*
Radix Angelicae Sinensis (*Dang Gui*), 4 *qian*
Rhizoma Carbonisata Zingiberis (*Hei Jiang*), 5 *fen*
Radix Praeparatus Glycyrrhizae (*Zhi Gan Cao*), 5 *fen*
Semen Pruni Persicae (*Tao Ren*), 10 pieces
Semen Nelumbinis Nuciferae (*Lian Zi*), 8 pieces

Decoct in water and take warm.

Jian Pi Li Shui Sheng Hua Tang (Fortify the Spleen, Disinhibit Water, Generating & Transforming Decoction) [Treats postpartum diarrhea with clots already eliminated]

Rhizoma Ligustici Wallichii (*Chuan Xiong*), 1 *qian*
Sclerotium Poriae Cocoris (*Fu Ling*), 1.5 *qian*

Radix Angelicae Sinensis (*Gui Shen*), 2 *qian*
Rhizoma Carbonisata Zingiberis (*Hei Jiang*), 4 *fen*
Pericarpium Citri Reticulatae (*Chen Pi*), 5 *fen*
Radix Praeparatus Glycyrrhizae (*Zhi Gan Cao*), 5 *fen*
Radix Panacis Ginseng (*Ren Shen*), 3 *qian*
Semen Myristicae Fragrantis (*Rou Guo*), 1 piece, processed
Rhizoma Atractylodis Macrocephalae (*Bai Zhu*), 1 *qian*, stir-fried
Rhizoma Alismatis (*Ze Xie*), 8 *fen*

In case of cold diarrhea, add 8 *fen* of Rhizoma Desiccata Zingiberis (*Gan Jiang*). In case of cold pain, add Fructus Seu Semen Amomi (*Sha Ren*) and Rhizoma Praeparata Zingiberis (*Pao Jiang*), each 8 *fen*. In case of hot diarrhea, add 8 *fen* of stir-fried Rhizoma Coptidis Chinensis (*Huang Lian*). In case of water diarrhea with abdominal pain and inability to transform (even) thin rice porridge, add Fructus Seu Semen Amomi 8 *fen*, and Fructus Germinatus Hordei Vulgaris (*Mai Ya*) and Fructus Crataegi (*Shan Zha*), each 1 *qian*. In case of diarrhea with acidic, putrefying foul smell, add Massa Medica Fermentata (*Shen Qu*) and Fructus Seu Semen Amomi (*Sha Ren*), each 8 *fen*. Persisting empty spleen qi with relief experienced only after diarrhea of what has (just) been taken in should be considered empty cold. In case of watery diarrhea, add 1 *qian* of Rhizoma Atractylodis (*Cang Zhu*) to dry dampness. In case of weak spleen qi and empty *yuan* or original qi, greatly supplementing is necessary in combination with food-dispersing, heat-clearing, and cold-eliminating medicinals as assistants. In case of severe weakness and form and complexion desertion, the first formula is the only choice and Radix Panacis Ginseng, Rhizoma Atractylodis Macrocephalae, Sclerotium Poriae Cocoris (*Fu Ling*), and Radix Praeparatus Aconiti Carmichaeli (*Fu Zi*) are indispensable medicinals. For all the types of diarrhea, add wine-fried Rhizoma Cimicifugae (*Sheng Ma*) and 10 pieces of Semen Nelumbinis Nuciferae (*Lian Zi*).

Wan Gu Bu Hua
Whole Grains Not Transformed
(*i.e.*, Undigested Food in the Stools)

(This is) caused by retarded transportation and conveyance due to postpartum taxation and fatigue injuring the spleen. It is called swill diarrhea. In addition, injury of the spleen and stomach due to overeating can cause the same (trouble). This is what is popularly known as *shui gu li* or water and grain dysentery. However, (if this occurs) less than three days after delivery when clots or lumps are not yet cleared or transformed, it is (due to) debilitated and weak spleen and stomach. Radix Panacis Ginseng (*Ren Shen*), Radix Astragali Seu Hedysari (*Huang Qi*), and Rhizoma Atractylodis Macrocephalae (*Bai Zhu*) should not be used for the time being. (Instead) simply administer *Sheng Hua Tang* plus Fructus Alpiniae Oxyphyllae (*Yi Zhi*), Radix Saussureae Seu Vladimiriae (*Mu Xiang*), and Fructus Seu Semen Amomi (*Sha Ren*) added to warm the spleen qi a little. After the clots or lumps are cleared, add Radix Panacis Ginseng, Radix Astragali Seu Hedysari, and Rhizoma Atractylodis Macrocephalae to supplement the qi; Semen Myristicae Fragrantis (*Rou Guo*), Radix Saussureae Seu Vladimiriae, Fructus Seu Semen Amomi, and Fructus Alpiniae Oxyphyllae (*Yi Zhi*) to warm the stomach; Rhizoma Cimicifugae (*Sheng Ma*) and Radix Bupleuri (*Chai Hu*) to clear stomach qi; and Rhizoma Alismatis (*Ze Xie*), Sclerotium Poriae Cocoris (*Fu Ling*), and Pericarpium Citri Reticulatae (*Chen Pi*) to disinhibit water. This is the best strategy.

Jia Wei Sheng Hua Tang (Added Flavors Generating & Transforming Decoction) [Treats untransformed food in stools less than three days after delivery when clots are not yet cleared]

Rhizoma Ligustici Wallichii (*Chuan Xiong*), 1 *qian*

Fructus Alpiniae Oxyphyllae (*Yi Zhi*), 1 *qian*
Radix Angelicae Sinensis (*Dang Gui*), 4 *qian*
Rhizoma Carbonisata Zingiberis (*Hei Jiang*), 4 *fen*
Radix Praeparatus Glycyrrhizae (*Zhi Gan Cao*), 4 *fen*
Semen Pruni Persicae (*Tao Ren*), 10 pieces
Sclerotium Poriae Cocoris (*Fu Ling*), 1.5 *qian*

[In a variant edition, Radix Angelicae Sinensis is 3 *qian* with 1 piece of Fructus Zizyphi Jujubae (*Zao*).]

Shen Ling Sheng Hua Tang (Ginseng & Poria Generating & Transforming Decoction) [Treats inability to transform food less than three days after delivery when clots are already cleared, a problem (actually) existing before pregnancy due to an originally weak condition]

Rhizoma Ligustici Wallichii (*Chuan Xiong*), 1 *qian*
Radix Angelicae Sinensis (*Dang Gui*), 2 *qian*
Rhizoma Carbonisata Zingiberis (*Hei Jiang*), 4 *fen*
Radix Praeparatus Glycyrrhizae (*Zhi Gan Cao*), 5 *fen*
Radix Panacis Ginseng (*Ren Shen*), 2 *qian*
Sclerotium Poriae Cocoris (*Fu Ling*), 1 *qian*
Radix Albus Paeoniae Lactiflorae (*Bai Shao*), 1 *qian*, stir-fried
Fructus Alpiniae Oxyphyllae (*Yi Zhi*), 1 *qian*, stir-fried
Rhizoma Atractylodis Macrocephalae (*Bai Zhu*), 2 *qian*, stir-fried with earth
Semen Myristicae Fragrantis (*Rou Guo*), 1 piece, processed

In case of diarrhea with much water, add Rhizoma Alismatis (*Ze Xie*) and Caulis Akebiae Mutong (*Mu Tong*), each 8 *fen*. In case of abdominal pain, add 8 *fen* of Fructus Seu Semen Amomi (*Sha Ren*). In case of thirst, add Tuber Ophiopogonis Japonicae (*Mai Dong*) and Fructus Schizandrae Chinensis (*Wu Wei Zi*). In case of cold diarrhea, add 1 *qian* of Rhizoma Carbonisata Zingiberis (*Hei Jiang*) and 4 *fen* of Radix Saussureae

Seu Vladimiriae (*Mu Xiang*). In case of food accumulation, add Massa Medica Fermentata (*Shen Qu*) and Fructus Germinatus Hordei Vulgaris (*Mai Ya*) to disperse grain food or Fructus Seu Semen Amomi and Fructus Crataegi (*Shan Zha*) to disperse meat food. In case of persisting postpartum diarrhea with empty, weak stomach qi and inability to transform food, it is proper to warm and assist the stomach qi by administering the *Liu Jun Zi Tang* (Six Gentlemen Decoction)[1] plus 4 *fen* of Radix Saussureae Seu Vladimiriae (*Mu Xiang*) and 1 piece of processed Semen Myristicae Fragrantis (*Rou Guo*).

[In a variant edition, there are 8 pieces of cored Semen Nelumbinis Nuciferae (*Lian Zi*) and 3 pieces of Fructus Zizyphi Jujubae (*Zao*).]

Li
Dysentery

Red and white dysentery with abdominal urgency, rectal heaviness, and frequent defecation contracted somewhere around the seventh day after delivery is most difficult to treat. If qi is regulated and blood moved in order to wipe out dysentery evils, worry is warranted that postpartum original qi may still be empty and weak. If *ying* or construction is enriched and qi boosted in order to greatly supplement (this) vacuity and weakness, then dysentery evils may be assisted. *Sheng Hua Tang* with Radix Saussureae Seu Vladimiriae (*Mu Xiang*) and Sclerotium Poriae Cocoris (*Fu Ling*) replacing Rhizoma Desiccata Zingiberis (*Gan Jiang*) is the only choice that

---

1 This formula consists of Radix Panacis Ginseng (*Ren Shen*), Rhizoma Atractylodis Macrocephalae (*Bai Zhu*), Sclerotium Poriae Cocoris (*Fu Ling*), Pericarpium Citri Reticulatae (*Chen Pi*), Rhizoma Pinelliae Ternatae (*Ban Xia*), and Radix Praeparatus Glycyrrhizae (*Zhi Gan Cao*).

is good at dispersing the lochia as well as curing dysentery, (accomplishing both) in a parallel and compatible way. Afterwards, one should administer *Xiang Lian Wan (Saussurea & Coptis Pills)*[2], in the hope that, if the condition gets better in 1-2 days, safety will be ensured. In case of empty dysentery and frequent diarrhea with brown, flowery stools and rectal heaviness contracted more than seven days after delivery, supplementation is undoubtedly needed in addition. If more than 20 days have passed since delivery and if the birthing woman is of strong constitution, it is proper to administer *Sheng Hua Tang* plus accumulation-moving medicinals such as Rhizoma Coptidis Chinensis (*Huang Lian*), Radix Scutellariae Baicalensis (*Huang Qin*), Cortex Magnoliae Officinalis (*Hou Po*), and Radix Albus Paeoniae Lactiflorae (*Shao Yao*).

Jia Jian Sheng Hua Tang (Modified Generating & Transforming Decoction) [Treats dysentery contracted within seven days after delivery]

Rhizoma Ligustici Wallichii (*Chuan Xiong*), 2 *qian*
Radix Angelicae Sinensis (*Dang Gui*), 5 *qian*
Radix Praeparatus Glycyrrhizae (*Zhi Gan Cao*), 5 *fen*
Semen Pruni Persicae (*Tao Ren*), 12 pieces
Sclerotium Poriae Cocoris (*Fu Ling*), 1 *qian*
Pericarpium Citri Reticulatae (*Chen Pi*), 4 *fen*
Radix Saussureae Seu Vladimiriae (*Mu Xiang*), ground, 3 *fen*

In case of red dysentery with abdominal pain, add 8 *fen* of Fructus Seu Semen Amomi (*Sha Ren*).

---

2 These pills are made by stir-frying 20 *liang* of Rhizoma Coptidis Chinensis (*Huang Lian*) together with 10 *liang* of Fructus Evodiae Rutecarpae (*Wu Zhu Yu*). Remove the Fructus Evodiae Rutecarpae and mix in 4 *liang*, 8 *qian* of Radix Saussureae Seu Vladimiriae (*Mu Xiang*) with the fried Rhizoma Coptidis Chinensis. Grind fine and make into pills with vinegar.

Qing Xue Wan (Green-Blue Blood Pills) [Treats dysentery with inability to eat]

Powder Radix Saussureae Seu Vladimiriae (*Mu Xiang*) and Rhizoma Coptidis Chinensis (*Huang Lian*) and mix with Pulvis Semenis Nelumbinis Nuciferae (*Lian Rou Fen*), each 1.5 *liang*. These should be mixed evenly and made into pills. Take 4 *qian* with wine.

Beyond three or four days after delivery, with clots cleared, 10 patterns may be given rise to when dysentery has been ameliorated a little. They are listed below and can be treated as instructed.

1. Postpartum persisting diarrhea: If the original qi has fallen with incontinence of defecation and the anus has seemingly prolapsed, it is appropriate to administer the *Liu Jun Zi Tang* (Six Gentlemen Decoction) plus 4 *fen* of Radix Saussureae Seu Vladimiriae (*Mu Xiang*), 1 piece of processed Semen Myristicae Fragrantis (*Rou Guo*), and 5 *fen* of Succus Zingiberis (*Jiang Zhi*).

2. Postpartum diarrhea and dysentery: If yellow in color, (indicating) vacuity and detriment of the true qi of spleen/earth, it is proper to administer *Bu Zhong Yi Qi Tang* (Supplement the Center, Boost the Qi Decoction) plus Radix Saussureae Seu Vladimiriae (*Mu Xiang*) and Semen Myristicae Fragrantis (*Rou Guo*).

3. Postpartum cereal (type) food injury: In case of diarrhea and dysentery, it is appropriate to administer *Sheng Hua Tang* plus Massa Medica Fermentata (*Shen Qu*) and Fructus Germinatus Hordei Vulgaris (*Mai Ya*).

[In a variant edition Massa Medica Fermentata and Fructus Germinatus Hordei Vulgaris are given at 1 *qian* each.]

4. Postpartum meat (type) food injury: In case of diarrhea and dysentery, it is proper to administer *Sheng Hua Tang* plus Fructus Crataegi (*Shan Zha*) and Fructus Seu Semen Amomi (*Sha Ren*).

5. Postpartum vacuity and weakness of stomach qi: In case of diarrhea and dysentery with untransformed food, it is necessary to warm and assist the stomach qi. (For this,) it is proper to administer *Liu Jun Zi Tang* plus 4 *fen* of Radix Saussureae Seu Vladimiriae (*Mu Xiang*) and 1 piece of processed Semen Myristicae Fragrantis (*Rou Guo*).

6. Postpartum vacuity and weakness of the spleen and stomach: In case of water swelling in the four limbs, it is proper to administer *Liu Jun Zi Tang* plus *Wu Pi San* (Five Skins Powder). [See *shui zhong* or water swelling in a later section.]

7. Postpartum diarrhea and dysentery: If there is no rectal heaviness but (the diarrhea) persists for a long time and will not stop, it is proper to administer *Liu Jun Zi Tang* plus Radix Saussureae Seu Vladimiriae (*Mu Xiang*) and Semen Myristicae Fragrantis (*Rou Guo*).

8. Postpartum red and white dysentery: In case of pain below the navel, (prescribe) Radix Angelicae Sinensis (*Dang Gui*), Cortex Magnoliae Officinalis (*Hou Po*), Rhizoma Coptidis Chinensis (*Huang Lian*), Semen Myristicae Fragrantis (*Rou Guo*), Radix Glycyrrhizae (*Gan Cao*), Semen Pruni Persicae (*Tao Ren*), and Rhizoma Ligustici Wallichii (*Chuan Xiong*).

9. Postpartum enduring dysentery: In case of red color, which is ascribed to blood vacuity, it is proper to administer *Si Wu Tang* (Four Ingredients Decoction) plus Herba Seu Flos

Schizonepetae Tenuifoliae (*Jing Jie*) and Radix Panacis Ginseng (*Ren Shen*).

10. Postpartum enduring dysentery: In case of white color, which is ascribed to qi vacuity, it is proper to administer *Liu Jun Zi Tang* plus Radix Saussureae Seu Vladimiriae (*Mu Xiang*) and Semen Myristicae Fragrantis (*Rou Guo*).

Huo Luan
Sudden Chaos (*i.e.*, Choleric Diseases)

If qi and blood are injured by taxation, the viscera and bowels become empty and vacuous, unable to transport or transform food. As the (combined) result of this and invasion of chill wind, ascension and descension of yin and yang become abnormal. The clear and turbid are disturbed within the spleen and stomach. Cold and heat are in disharmony and evil and righteous are in conflict. (Therefore,) above and below are plunged into sudden turmoil.

Sheng Hua Liu He Tang (Generating & Transforming Six Harmonies Decoction) [Treats postpartum choleric disease with blood clots not yet cleared up]

Rhizoma Ligustici Wallichii (*Chuan Xiong*), 2 *qian*
Radix Angelicae Sinensis (*Dang Gui*), 4 *qian*
Rhizoma Carbonisata Zingiberis (*Hei Jiang*)
Radix Praeparatus Glycyrrhizae (*Zhi Gan Cao*)
Pericarpium Citri Reticulatae (*Chen Pi*)
Herba Agastachis Seu Pogostemi (*Huo Xiang*), each 4 *fen*
Fructus Seu Semen Amomi (*Sha Ren*), 6 *fen*
Sclerotium Poriae Cocoris (*Fu Ling*), 1 *qian*
Rhizoma Recens Zingiberis (*Sheng Jiang*), 3 slices

Decoct.

Fu Zi San (Aconite Powder) [Treats postpartum choleric disease with vomiting, diarrhea, and counterflow chilling of the limbs. It can be administered only after clot or lump pain has disappeared.]

Rhizoma Atractylodis Macrocephalae (*Bai Zhu*), 1 *qian*
Radix Angelicae Sinensis (*Dang Gui*), 2 *qian*
Pericarpium Citri Reticulatae (*Chen Pi*)
Rhizoma Carbonisata Zingiberis (*Hei Jiang*)
Flos Caryophylii (*Ding Xiang*)
Radix Glycyrrhizae (*Gan Cao*), each 4 *fen*

Grind into powder. Take 2 *qian* with porridge.

[In a variant edition there is 5 *fen* of Radix Praeparatus Aconiti Carmichaeli (*Fu Zi*).]

Wen Zhong Tang (Warm the Center Decoction) [Treats postpartum choleric disease with incessant vomiting and diarrhea. It is prescribed in the absence of clot or lump pain.]

Radix Panacis Ginseng (*Ren Shen*), 1 *qian*
Rhizoma Atractylodis Macrocephalae (*Bai Zhu*), 1.5 *qian*
Radix Angelicae Sinensis (*Dang Gui*), 2 *qian*
Cortex Magnoliae Officinalis (*Hou Po*), 8 *fen*
Rhizoma Carbonisata Zingiberis (*Hei Jiang*), 4 *fen*
Sclerotium Poriae Cocoris (*Fu Ling*), 1 *qian*
Semen Alpiniae Katsumadai (*Cao Dou Kou*), 6 *fen*
Rhizoma Recens Zingiberis (*Sheng Jiang*), 3 slices

Decoct in water and take.

Ou Ni Bu Shi
Counterflow Retching (&) Inability to Eat

After delivery, if the viscera and bowels are injured by taxation, cold evils will find it easy to overwhelm the spleen and stomach, resulting in counterflow qi retching and vomiting with inability to eat. There are also cases of retching due to not yet cleared static blood as well as cases of retching due to unclear stomach openings because of entry of phlegm qi into the stomach. These should be balanced according to the condition.

Jia Jian Sheng Hua Tang (Modified Generating & Transforming Decoction) [Treats counterflow retching with inability to eat in birthing women]

Rhizoma Ligustici Wallichii (*Chuan Xiong*), 1 *qian*
Radix Angelicae Sinensis (*Dang Gui*), 3 *qian*
Rhizoma Carbonisata Zingiberis (*Hei Jiang*)
Fructus Seu Semen Amomi (*Sha Ren*)
Herba Agastachis Seu Pogostemi (*Huo Xiang*), each 5 *fen*
Caulis Bambusae In Taeniis (*Dan Zhu Ye*), 7 leaves

Decoct in water and take with 2 spoons of Succus Zingiberis (*Jiang Zhi*).

Wen Wei Ding Xiang San (Warm the Stomach Clove Powder) [Treats counterflow retching and inability to eat beyond seven days after delivery]

Radix Angelicae Sinensis (*Dang Gui*), 3 *qian*
Rhizoma Atractylodis Macrocephalae (*Bai Zhu*), 2 *qian*
Rhizoma Carbonisata Zingiberis (*Hei Jiang*), 4 *fen*
Flos Caryophylli (*Ding Xiang*), 4 *fen*
Radix Panacis Ginseng (*Ren Shen*), 1 *qian*

Pericarpium Citri Reticulatae (*Chen Pi*), 5 *fen*
Radix Praeparatus Glycyrrhizae (*Zhi Gan Cao*), 5 *fen*
Radix Peucedani (*Qian Hu*), 5 *fen*
Herba Agastachis Seu Pogostemi (*Huo Xiang*), 5 *fen*
Rhizoma Recens Zingiberis (*Sheng Jiang*), 3 slices

Decoct in water and take.

Shi Lian San (Lotus Seed Powder) [Treats retching and vomiting, surging into the heart, and visual dizziness in birthing women]

Semen Nelumbinis Nuciferae (*Shi Lian Zi*), peeled, cored, 1.5 *liang*
Sclerotium Poriae Cocoris (*Bai Fu Ling*), 1 *liang*
Flos Caryophylli (*Ding Xiang*), 5 *fen*

Grind into a fine powder and take with thin rice porridge.

[In a variant edition there is Rhizoma Atractylodis Macrocephalae (*Bai Zhu*) instead of Sclerotium Poriae Cocoris. Flos Caryophylli is 5 *qian*. The physician can use his own discretion.]

Sheng Jin Yi Ye Tang (Generate Fluids, Boost Humor Decoction) [Treats thirst with shortness of breath in weak and empty birthing women. These are due to postpartum scant blood, profuse sweating, and interior vexation failing to generate fluids and humor.]

Radix Panacis Ginseng (*Ren Shen*)
Tuber Ophiopogonis Japonicae (*Mai Dong*), cored
Sclerotium Poriae Cocoris (*Fu Ling*), each 1 *liang*
Fructus Zizyphi Jujubae (*Da Zao*)
Herba Lophatheri Gracilis (*Zhu Ye*)

Fructus Levis Tritici (*Fu Xiao Mai*)
Radix Praeparatus Glycyrrhizae (*Zhi Gan Cao*)
Ramulus Trichosanthis Kirlowii (*Gua Lou Geng*)

In case of constant severe thirst, add Rhizoma Phragmitis Communis (*Lu Geng*).

[In a variant edition Radix Panacis Ginseng is (given at) 1 *qian*; Tuber Ophiopogonis Japonicae and Sclerotium Poriae Cocoris, 3 *qian*.]

Ke Sou
Coughing

In the treatment of external invasion of wind cold within seven days after delivery with cough, nasal congestion, heavy voice, and aversion to cold, do not use *Ma Huang Tang* to promote perspiration. In case of coughing with lateral costal pain, do not use *Chai Hu Tang* (Bupleurum Decoction). In case of coughing with rales, little phlegm, and a red facial complexion, do not use cooling medicinals. For either fire coughing or phlegm coughing in postpartum cases, no cooling medicinals should be used till after half a month of balancing and regulating. In no case should they be used earlier than that.

Jia Wei Sheng Hua Tang (Added Flavors Generating & Transforming Decoction) [Treats postpartum external invasion of wind cold with coughing, nasal congestion, and heavy voice]

Rhizoma Ligustici Wallichii (*Chuan Xiong*), 1 *qian*
Radix Angelicae Sinensis (*Dang Gui*), 2 *qian*
Semen Pruni Armeniacae (*Xing Ren*), 10 pieces
Radix Platycodi Grandiflori (*Jie Geng*), 4 *fen*
Rhizoma Anemarrhenae (*Zhi Mu*), 8 *fen*

In case of phlegm, add Massa Medica Fermentata Cum Pinelliam (*Ban Xia Qu*). In case of vacuity, weakness, sweating, and coughing, add Radix Panacis Ginseng (*Ren Shen*). In a word, diaphoresis is prohibited postpartum.

[In a variant version Rhizoma Anemarrhenae (is given at) 4 *fen*.]

Jia Shen An Fei Sheng Hua Tang (Added Ginseng Calm the Lungs Generating & Transforming Decoction) [Treats postpartum vacuity and weakness with external invasion of wind cold within 10 days after delivery with coughing, heavy voice, and phlegm or body heat (*i.e.*, generalized fever), headache, and profuse sweating.]

Rhizoma Ligustici Wallichii (*Chuan Xiong*), 1 *qian*
Radix Panacis Ginseng (*Ren Shen*), 1 *qian*
Rhizoma Anemarrhenae (*Zhi Mu*), 1 *qian*
Cortex Mori Albi (*Sang Bai Pi*), 1 *qian*
Radix Angelicae Sinensis (*Dang Gui*), 2 *qian*
Semen Pruni Armeniacae (*Xing Ren*), 10 pieces, skinned & tip-nipped
Radix Glycyrrhizae (*Gan Cao*), 4 *fen*
Radix Platycodi Grandiflori (*Jie Geng*), 4 *fen*
Rhizoma Pinelliae Ternatae (*Ban Xia*), 7 *fen*
Exocarpium Citri Reticulatae (*Ju Hong*), 3 *fen*

For an empty patient with much phlegm, add 1 cup of Succus Bambusae (*Zhu Li*) and half a spoonful of Succus Zingiberis (*Jiang Zhi*).

[Note: In the discussion on coughing (given above), it is clearly stated that even in case of fire coughing, cool medicinals should not be used unscrupulously earlier than half a month after (delivery), and this admonition is made in a rigid way.

However, in both the first and the second formulas (given above), there is Rhizoma Anemarrhenae. The note inserted in small characters (*i.e.*, inserted by an earlier editor, reading) "external invasion of wind cold" must imply that after such invasion, dryness and heat are already brewed. Consequently, (Rhizoma Anemarrhenae) is used as a last resort. However, this implication is not (adequately) brought out in that note. If this were not the case and such a cool medicinal were (meant) to be used immediately following (external) invasion, these formulas and this discussion would be like a square peg in a round hole. The reader should try to well understand the subtle undertones of (our) predecessors. Then one can avoid (the fault of) applying old formulas without weighing (their propriety).

Jia Wei Si Wu Tang (Added Flavors 4 Ingredient Decoction) [Treats dry coughing with rales and little phlegm more than half a month after delivery]

Rhizoma Ligustici Wallichii (*Chuan Xiong*)
Radix Albus Paeoniae Lactiflorae (*Bai Shao*)
Rhizoma Anemarrhenae (*Zhi Mu*)
Semen Trichosanthis Kirlowii (*Gua Lou Ren*), each 1 *qian*
Radix Rehmanniae (*Di Huang*)
Radix Angelicae Sinensis (*Dang Gui*), each 2 *qian*
Fructus Terminaliae Chebulae (*Ke Zi*), 2 *qian*
Flos Tussilagi Farfarae (*Dong Hua*), 6 *fen*
Radix Platycodi Grandiflori (*Jie Geng*), 4 *fen*
Radix Glycyrrhizae (*Gan Cao*), 4 *fen*
Fructus Aristolochiae (*Dou Ling*), 4 *fen*
Rhizoma Recens Zingiberis (*Jiang*), 1 large slice

Shui Zhong
Water Swelling

Postpartum water qi (manifested by) edematous swelling of the hands and feet with bright, shiny skin complexion is due to vacuity of the spleen failing to restrain water and vacuity of the kidneys failing to move water. Priority must be given to greatly supplementing the qi and blood with the use of Rhizoma Atractylodis (*Cang Zhu*), Rhizoma Atractylodis Macrocephalae (*Bai Zhu*), and Sclerotium Poriae Cocoris (*Fu Ling*) as assistants to supplementing the spleen. Stoppage and fullness require the use of Pericarpium Citri Reticulatae (*Chen Pi*), Rhizoma Pinelliae Ternatae (*Ban Xia*), and Rhizoma Cyperi Rotundi (*Xiang Fu*) to disperse (them). For empty patients, add Radix Panacis Ginseng (*Ren Shen*) and Caulis Akebiae Mu Tong (*Mu Tong*). In case of heat, add Radix Scutellariae Baicalensis (*Huang Qin*) and Tuber Ophiopogonis Japonicae (*Mai Dong*) to clear lung/metal. To fortify the spleen and disinhibit water, (use) *Bu Zhong Yi Qi Tang*. (If) more than 7 days (after delivery), add Radix Panacis Ginseng, Rhizoma Atractylodis Macrocephalae, each 2 *qian*; Sclerotium Poriae Cocoris and Radix Albus Paeoniae Lactiflorae (*Bai Shao*), each 1 *qian*; Pericarpium Citri Reticulatae, 5 *fen*; Fructus Chaenomelis Lagenariae (*Mu Gua*), 8 *fen*; Fructus Perillae Frutescentis (*Zi Su*), Caulis Akebiae Mutong (*Mu Tong*), Pericarpium Arecae Catechu (*Da Fu Pi*), Rhizoma Atractylodis, and Cortex Magnoliae Officinalis (*Hou Po*), each 4 *fen*. In case of constipation, add Semen Pruni (*Yu Li Ren*) and Semen Cannabis Sativae (*Ma Ren*), each 1 qian. In case of swelling with absence of sweating due to injury of the spleen by cold evils and damp qi, it is proper to add Cortex Zingiberis (*Jiang Pi*), Rhizoma Pinelliae Ternatae (*Ban Xia*), and Folium Perillae Frutescentis (*Su Ye*) to a qi-supplementing formula in order to exteriorize sweat.

Wu Pi San (Five Skins Powder) [Treats postpartum water swelling of the face and eyes, swelling and distention of the four limbs, dyspnea due to wind damp invading and injuring the spleen, and congealed and stagnated qi and blood]

Radix Acanthopanacis (*Wu Jia Pi*)
Cortex Radicis Lycii (*Di Gu Pi*)
Pericarpium Arecae Catechu (*Da Fu Pi*)
Cortex Sclerotii Poriae Cocoris (*Fu Ling Pi*), each 1 *qian*
Cortex Zingiberis (*Jiang Pi*), 1 *qian*
Fructus Zizyphi Jujubae (*Zao*), 1 piece

Decoct in water and take.

In addition, it is stated that after delivery, if it is not cleared up, the lochia will be retained in the *bao lou* or connecting vessels of the uterus resulting in water swelling. It is wrong to treat this as water qi and prescribe such medicinals as Radix Euphorbiae Kansui (*Gan Sui*). Administer only *Tiao Jing San* (Balance the Menses Powder) and blood will be moved and swelling dispersed.

Tiao Jing San (Balance the Menses Powder)

Myrrha (*Mo Yao*), ground separately
Succinum (*Hu Po*), ground separately, each 1 *qian*
Cortex Cinnamomi (*Rou Gui*)
Radix Rubrus Paeoniae Lactiflorae (*Chi Shao*)
Radix Angelicae Sinensis (*Dang Gui*), each 1 *qian*

Powder finely the above. Each time take 5 *fen*. Take with a small amount of Succus Zingiberis (*Jiang Zhi*) mixed with wine.

[This formula is able to balance the menses and treats abdominal pain.]

Liu Zhu
Flowing, Pouring (Sore)

After delivery, the lochia may flow into the joints of the lumbar region, arms, and feet giving rise to diffuse swellings or knotted lumps. If this lingers long, the swelling will exaggerate, causing pain and fatigue of the body and limbs. It is necessary to immediately perform the onion-ironing method to externally treat the swelling. Internally, administer *Shen Gui Sheng Hua Tang* (Ginseng & Dang Gui Generating & Transforming Decoction) to disperse blood stagnation. This allows for no delay. The mature (swelling) will be dispersed, while the immature will break.

Cong Yun Fa (Onion-ironing Method)

Heat a handful of Chinese green onion, smash, and make this into a cake. Apply this to the painful area. Cover with 2-3 layers of cloth and then iron it.

Shen Gui Sheng Hua Tang (Ginseng & Dang Gui Generating & Transforming Decoction)

Rhizoma Ligustici Wallichii (*Chuan Xiong*), 1.5 *qian*
Radix Angelicae Sinensis (*Dang Gui*), 2 *qian*
Radix Praeparatus Glycyrrhizae (*Zhi Gan Cao*), 5 *fen*
Radix Panacis Ginseng (*Ren Shen*), 1.2 *qian*
Radix Astragali Seu Hedysari (*Huang Qi*), 1.5 *qian*
Cortex Cinnamomi (*Rou Gui*), 5 *fen*
Lignum Aquilariae Agallochae (*Ma Ti Xiang*), 2 *qian*

Unless qi and blood are supplemented, a disciplined diet is kept, and care is taken about the daily life, no survival can be expected. If the swelling has become enlarged and painful but daily life activities and appetite are not affected, the disease qi has not (yet) penetrated deep and form qi has not yet been injured. This is easy to cure. Diffuse swelling with slight pain, fatigue arising on movement, and insufficient food intake is most difficult to cure. In case of nondevelopment of pus or failure (of the swelling) to rupture (due to) qi and blood vacuity, it is proper to administer *Ba Zhen Tang* (Eight Pearls Decoction). In case of abhorrence of and aversion to cold (due to) yang qi vacuity, it is proper to administer *Shi Quan Da Bu Wan* (Ten Complete Great Supplementing Pills).[3] In case of great heat following supplementation (due to) yin (&) blood vacuity, it is proper to administer the *Si Wu Tang* (Four Ingredient Decoction) with Radix Panacis Ginseng (*Ren Shen*), Rhizoma Atractylodis Macrocephalae (*Bai Zhu*), and Cortex Radicis Moutan (*Dan Pi*). In case of counterflow retching (due to) stomach qi vacuity, it is proper to administer *Liu Jun Zi Tang* (Six Gentlemen Decoction) with Rhizoma Praeparata Zingiberis (*Pao Jiang*) and Rhizoma Desiccata Zingiberis (*Gan Jiang*). In case of low food intake and generalized fatigue (due to) spleen qi vacuity, it is proper to administer the *Bu Zhong Yi Qi Tang* (Supplement the Center, Boost the Qi Decoction). In case of counterflow chilling of the four limbs and frequent urination (due to) kidney qi vacuity, (administer) *Bu Zhong Yi Qi Tang* plus 1 qian of Fructus Alpiniae Oxyphyllae (*Yi Zhi*). *Shen Xian Hui Dong San* (The Immortal Returning to his Cave Abode Powder)[4] is (a remedy) to treat postpartum streaming

---

3 The ingredients of this formula include Radix Astragali Seu Hedysari (*Huang Qi*), Cortex Cinnamomi (*Rou Gui*), Radix Panacis Ginseng (*Ren Shen*), Radix Coquitus Rehmanniae (*Shu Di*), Rhizoma Atractylodis Macrocephalae (*Bai Zhu*), Radix Angelicae Sinensis (*Dang Gui*), Radix Albus Paeoniae Lactiflorae (*Bai Shao*), Rhizoma Ligustici Wallichii (*Chuan Xiong*), Sclerotium Poriae Cocoris (*Fu Ling*), Radix Praeparatus Glycyrrhizae (*Zhi Gan Cao*).

4 This formula is composed of Radix Albus Paeoniae Lactiflorae (*Bai Shao*), 3 qian; Radix Angelicae Sinensis (*Dang Gui*), Cortex Cinnamomi (*Rou Gui*), Radix Glycyrrhizae (*Gan Cao*), Pericarpium Citri Reticulatae (*Chen Pi*), Radix Panacis

lochia which has been retained long enough to result in swelling. It is appropriate to use in order to conduct pus, but it should not be used if qi and blood are effulgent without supplementation.

Peng Zhang
Inflation (&) Distention

The patient was weak in the past and, in addition, has been taxed in the course of labor. (Now) central qi is insufficient, the chest and diaphragm are inhibited, and conveyance and transportation are retarded. If *Sheng Hua Tang* is administered upon finishing labor to disperse clots and stop pain and *Jia Shen Sheng Hua Tang* is administered in addition to fortify the spleen and stomach, this condition of fullness in the center can never occur. Inflation and distention are caused by misapplication of dispersing in case of food injury and dissipating in case of qi depression and by retention of the lochia due to overeating chilly foods. This distention is further exacerbated by misapplication of precipitating in case of dry, bound stools due to empty blood. It should be understood that, after blood clots are cleared, dual vacuity of the qi and blood requires greatly supplementing the qi and blood to supplement vacuity of the center. If the physician knows no more than that dispersing is appropriate for food injury, that dissipating is appropriate for qi depression, that the lochia requires attacking, and that constipation calls for precipitation, then the stomach qi will be erroneously damaged, fullness and oppression will get worse, and the qi will be stopped from ascending

---

Ginseng (*Ren Shen*), Rhizoma Atractylodis Macrocephalae (*Bai Zhu*), and Radix Astragali Seu Hedysari (*Huang Qi*), each 1 liang; Radix Coquitus Rehmanniae (*Shu Di*), Fructus Schizandrae Chinensis (*Wu Wei Zi*), and Sclerotium Poriae Cocoris (*Fu Ling*), each 7.5 qian; and Radix Polygalae Tenuifoliae (*Yuan Zhi*), 5 qian. These should be mixed and ground. Dosage is 4 *qian*.

and descending. When damp heat accumulates over a long period of time, inflation and distention result. One should understand that, (in postpartum cases,) if abducting dispersion is realized through supplementation of the center, the spleen and the stomach will be made strong, while the food qi causing injury will be dispersed and dissipated. If blood is assisted and simultaneously moved, defecation will automatically be freed and the lochia automatically moved.

If, in the case of postpartum windstroke and insufficiency of qi, slight fullness has developed into distention as a result of misapplication of qi-consuming medicinals, administer ***Bu Zhong Yi Qi Tang.***

Radix Panacis Ginseng (*Ren Shen*), 5 *fen*
Radix Angelicae Sinensis (*Dang Gui*), 5 *fen*
Rhizoma Atractylodis Macrocephalae (*Bai Zhu*), 5 *fen*
Sclerotium Poriae Cocoris (*Bai Fu Ling*), 1 *qian*
Rhizoma Ligustici Wallichii (*Chuan Xiong*), 4 *fen*
Radix Albus Paeoniae Lactiflorae (*Bai Shao*), 4 *fen*
Semen Raphani Sativi (*Luo Bo Zi*), 4 *fen*
Radix Saussureae Seu Vladimiriae (*Mu Xiang*), 3 *fen*

[In a variant edition Radix Panacis Ginseng and Rhizoma Atractylodis Macrocephalae (are given at) 1 *qian* and Radix Angelicae Sinensis at 2 *qian*. Also, there is 1 slice of Rhizoma Recens Zingiberis (*Jiang*).]

If food injury has developed into distention or accumulation of lumps in the lateral costal region as a result of misapplication of abducting dispersion, it is proper to administer ***Jian Pi Tang*** (Fortify the Spleen Decoction)

Radix Panacis Ginseng (*Ren Shen*)
Rhizoma Atractylodis Macrocephalae (*Bai Zhu*)

Radix Angelicae Sinensis (*Dang Gui*), each 3 *qian*
Sclerotium Poriae Cocoris (*Bai Fu Ling*)
Radix Albus Paeoniae Lactiflorae (*Bai Shao*)
Massa Medica Fermentata (*Shen Qu*)
Fructus Evodiae Rutecarpae (*Wu Yu*), each 1 *qian*
Fructus Seu Semen Amomi (*Sha Ren*)
Fructus Germinatus Hordei Vulgaris (*Mai Ya*), each 5 *fen*

[In a variant edition Radix Panacis Ginseng and Rhizoma Atractylodis Macrocephalae (are given at) 2 *qian*.]

If constipation has developed into distention with abdominal pain as a result of misapplication of precipitating medicinals, it is proper to administer ***Yang Rong Sheng Hua Tang*** (Nurture Construction Generating & Transforming Decoction)

Radix Angelicae Sinensis (*Dang Gui*), 4 *qian*
Radix Albus Paeoniae Lactiflorae (*Bai Shao*), 1 *qian*
Sclerotium Poriae Cocoris (*Bai Fu Ling*), 1 *qian*
Radix Panacis Ginseng (*Ren Shen*), 1 *qian*
Rhizoma Atractylodis Macrocephalae (*Bai Zhu*), 2 *qian*
Pericarpium Citri Reticulatae (*Chen Pi*), 5 *fen*
Pericarpium Arecae Catechu (*Da Fu Pi*), 5 *fen*
Rhizoma Cyperi Rotundi (*Xiang Fu*), 5 *fen*
Herba Cistanchis (*Cong Rong*), 1 *qian*
Semen Pruni Persicae (*Tao Ren*), 10 pieces, processed

In case of clot or lump pain, take (the above) with *Si Xiao Wan* (Four Dispersing Pills).[5] (In case of) repeated inappropriate precipitating, it is proper to administer half a *jin* of Radix Panacis Ginseng (*Ren Shen*) and Radix Angelicae Sinensis (*Dang Gui*).

---

5 The ingredients of this formula are unknown.

[In a variant edition there is no Semen Pruni Persicae.]

Zheng Chong Jing Ji
Racing Heart (&) Fright Palpitations

As a result of worry, fright, taxation, fatigue, and loss of much blood in the course of delivery, the heart jumps and beats and is not calm. This is called *zheng chong* or racing of the heart. Hypersensitivity with liability to shock and fright in addition to a timorous heart as if fearing arrest are called *jing ji* or fright palpitations. To treat either of the two disorders, there is no other choice but to harmonize the spleen and stomach. When the *zhi* or orientation becomes tranquil and the spirit becomes clear, this disease is cured. Before postpartum blood clots are eliminated, it is proper to administer *Sheng Hua Tang* to supplement the blood as well as to move the clots. When the blood is made effulgent, the racing (of the heart) will become tranquil and fright (palpitations) will become level. (Thus,) there is no need to add spirit-calming or orientation-stabilizing formulas. If these troubles arise after clots are eliminated and pain is relieved, it is proper to administer ***Jia Jian Yang Rong Tang*** (Modified Nurture Construction Decoction).

Radix Angelicae Sinensis (*Dang Gui*), 2 *qian*
Rhizoma Ligustici Wallichii (*Chuan Xiong*), 2 *qian*
Sclerotium Pararadicis Poriae Cocoris (*Fu Shen*), 1 *qian*
Radix Panacis Ginseng (*Ren Shen*), 1 *qian*
Semen Zizyphi Spinosae (*Zao Ren*), 1 *qian*, stir-fried
Tuber Ophiopogonis Japonicae (*Mai Dong*), 1 *qian*
Radix Polygalae Tenuifoliae (*Yuan Zhi*), 1 *qian*
Rhizoma Atractylodis Macrocephalae (*Bai Zhu*), 1 *qian*
Radix Praeparatus Astragali Seu Hedysari (*Zhi Huang Qi*), 1 *qian*
Arillus Euphoriae Longanae (*Yuan Rou*), 8 pieces
Pericarpium Citri Reticulatae (*Chen Pi*), 4 *fen*

Radix Praeparatus Glycyrrhizae (*Zhi Cao*), 4 *fen*
Rhizoma Recens Zingiberis (*Jiang*)

Decoct.

In case of empty vexation, add Succus Bambusae (*Zhu Li*) and Succus Zingiberis (*Jiang Zhi*), subtract Rhizoma Ligustici Wallichii and Tuber Ophiopogonis Japonicae, and then add again 1 ball of Caulis Bambusae In Taeniis (*Zhu Ru*). If Radix Saussureae Seu Vladimiriae (*Mu Xiang*) is added, the formula becomes *Gui Pi Tang* (Return the Spleen Decoction).

Yang Xin Tang (Nurture the Heart Decoction) [Treats postpartum disturbed heart blood and restless heart spirit]

Radix Praeparatus Astragali Seu Hedysari (*Zhi Huang Qi*), 1 *qian*
Sclerotium Pararadicis Poriae Cocoris (*Fu Shen*), 8 *fen*
Rhizoma Ligustici Wallichii (*Chuan Xiong*), 8 *fen*
Radix Angelicae Sinensis (*Dang Gui*), 2 *qian*
Tuber Ophiopogonis Japonicae (*Mai Dong*), 1.8 *qian*
Radix Polygalae Tenuifoliae (*Yuan Zhi*), 8 *fen*
Semen Biotae Orientalis (*Bai Zi Ren*), 1 *qian*
Radix Panacis Ginseng (*Ren Shen*), 1.5 *qian*
Radix Praeparatus Glycyrrhizae (*Zhi Cao*), 4 *fen*
Fructus Schizandrae Chinensis (*Wu Wei*), 10 pieces
Rhizoma Recens Zingiberis (*Jiang*)

Decoct in water and take.

[In a variant edition there are (also) 6 pieces of Arillus Euphoriae Longanae (*Yuan Rou*).]

Gu Zheng
Steaming Bone

It is proper to administer *Bao Zhen Tang* (Protect the True Decoction) (for this condition). Prior to it, administer *Qing Gu San* (Clear the Bones Powder).[6]

Chai Hu Mei Lian Tang (Bupleurum, Peucedanum, Coptis, & Mume Decoction) [Offers rapid effect if taken with decocted *Qing Gu San*]

Radix Bupleuri (*Chai Hu*)
Radix Peucedani (*Qian Hu*)
Rhizoma Coptidis Chinensis (*Huang Lian*)
Fructus Pruni Mume (*Wu Mei*), pitted

Each 2 *liang*, powdered for use. Obtain 1 pig's spine, 1 pig's gallbladder, and 10 white sections of leek stalk, 1 *cun* each. Crush these together, mix with 1 wine-cupful of child's urine, and stir into a thin paste. Add the powdered medicinals and pound again. Make pills the size of mung beans. Take 30-40 pills each time with boiled water. In case of abundant heat above the diaphragm, take these after meals. This formula can be used for steaming bones in both men and women and is not merely specific to birthing women.

Bao Zhen Tang (Protect the True Decoction)

Radix Astragali Seu Hedysari (*Huang Qi*), 6 *fen*

---

6 This formula is composed of Radix Stellariae Dichotomae (*Yin Chai Hu*), 1.5 *qian*; Rhizoma Coptidis Chinensis (*Huang Lian*), Radix Gentianae Macrophyllae (*Qin Jiao*), Carapax Amydae (*Bei Jia*), Cortex Radicis Lycii (*Di Gu Pi*), Herba Artemesiae Apiaceae (*Qing Hao*), Rhizoma Anemarrhenae (*Zhi Mu*), each 1 *qian*; and Radix Glycyrrhizae (*Gan Cao*), 5 *fen*.

Radix Panacis Ginseng (*Ren Shen*), 2 *qian*
Rhizoma Atractylodis Macrocephalae (*Bai Zhu*), 2 *qian*, stir-fried
Radix Praeparatus Glycyrrhizae (*Zhi Cao*), 4 *fen*
Rhizoma Ligustici Wallichii (*Chuan Xiong*), 6 *fen*
Radix Angelicae Sinensis (*Dang Gui*), 2 *qian*
Tuber Asparagi Cochinensis (*Tian Dong*), 1 *qian*
Tuber Ophiopogonis Japonicae (*Mai Dong*), 2 *qian*
Radix Albus Paeoniae Lactiflorae (*Bai Shao*), 2 *qian*
Fructus Lycii Chinensis (*Gou Qi*), 2 *qian*
Rhizoma Coptidis Chinensis (*Huang Lian*), 6 *fen*, stir-fried
Cortex Phellodendri (*Huang Bai*), 6 *fen*, stir-fried
Rhizoma Anemarrhenae (*Zhi Mu*), 2 *qian*
Radix Rehmanniae (*Sheng Di*), 2 *qian*
Fructus Schizandrae Chinensis (*Wu Wei*), 10 pieces
Cortex Radicis Lycii (*Di Gu Pi*), 6 *fen*
Fructus Zizyphi Jujubae (*Zao*), 3 pieces, pitted

Decoct in water and take.

[In a variant edition there is no Tuber Ophiopogonis Japonicae or Rhizoma Coptidis Chinensis.]

Jia Wei Da Zao Wan (Added Flavors Great Creation Pills) [Treats steaming bone taxation fever. Administer this formula if *Qing Gu San* and *(Chai Hu) Mei Lian Wan* have failed to bring effect.]

Radix Panacis Ginseng (*Ren Shen*), 1 *liang*
Radix Angelicae Sinensis (*Dang Gui*), 1 *liang*
Tuber Ophiopogonis Japonicae (*Mai Dong*), 8 *fen*
Herba Dendrobii (*Shi Hu*), 8 *fen*, steamed with wine
Radix Bupleuri (*Chai Hu*), 6 *qian*
Radix Rehmanniae (*Sheng Di*), 2 *liang*
Rhizoma Coptidis Chinensis (*Huang Lian*), 5 *qian*
Radix Dioscoreae Oppositae (*Shan Yao*), 1 *liang*

Fructus Lycii Chinensis (*Gou Qi*), 1 *liang*
Cortex Phellodendri (*Huang Bai*), 7 *fen*, stir-fried

First smash the Tuber Ophiopogonis Japonicae and Radix Rehmanniae together. Then mix these with the rest of the medicinals and pound again. Shape the mixture in pills. Besides, steam and then pound Placentis Hominis (*He Che*). Then bake and prepare into pills with heated honey.

[In a variant edition Tuber Ophiopogonis Japonicae and Herba Dendrobii (are given at) 8 *qian;* Radix Bupleuri at 5 *qian;* and Cortex Phellodendri, stir-fried with wine, at 4 *fen.*]

Xin Tong
Heart Pain

This is pain in the stomach venter or *wei wan*. It is caused by taxation injury, wind cold, and eating cold foods. Because the venter is situated below the heart, the pain is popularly known as heart pain. How can the heart be painful? When blood is insufficient, there occurs racing of the heart and fright palpitations with restlessness. Once the heart is really painful, the hands and feet must exhibit a green-blue, cyanotic or black complexion and death is impending. The appropriate treatment is to dissipate the cold qi and disperse the cold substance in the stomach. *Sheng Hua Tang* is immediately needed with medicinals to disperse cold food as assistants. Then, cure is ensured without fail. If no blood lumps are found through inquiry, dull pain which is relievable by pressure should be diagnosed as empty (pain) and treated by supplementation. Postpartum heart and abdominal pain are similar. If cold food and qi go up and attack the heart, there arises heart pain. If they go down and attack the abdomen, there arises abdominal pain. In either case, administer *Sheng Hua Tang* with warming and dissipating medicinals such as Cortex Cinnamomi (*Rou Gui*) and Fructus Evodiae Rutecarpae (*Wu Yu*) added.

Jia Wei Sheng Hua Tang (Added Flavors Generating & Transforming Decoction)

Rhizoma Ligustici Wallichii (*Chuan Xiong*), 1 *qian*
Radix Angelicae Sinensis (*Dang Gui*), 3 *qian*
Rhizoma Carbonisata Zingiberis (*Hei Jiang*), 5 *fen*
Cortex Cinnamomi (*Rou Gui*), 8 *fen*
Fructus Evodiae Rutecarpae (*Wu Yu*), 8 *fen*
Fructus Seu Semen Amomi (*Sha Ren*), 8 *fen*
Radix Praeparatus Glycyrrhizae (*Zhi Cao*), 5 *fen*

In case of cold food injury, add Cortex Cinnamomi and Fructus Evodiae Rutecarpae. In case of cereal (type) food injury, add Massa Medica Fermentata (*Shen Qu*) and Fructus Germinatus Hordei Vulgaris (*Mai Ya*). In case of meat (type) food injury, add Fructus Crataegi (*Shan Zha*) and Fructus Seu Semen Amomi. In case of constipation, add Herba Cistanchis (*Rou Cong Rong*).

Fu Tong
Abdominal Pain

First of all, enquire about the presence or absence of clots. If there is clot or lump pain, only administer *Sheng Hua Tang* plus 2 qian of *Shi Xiao San* (Laugh-exciting Powder) mixed in (after decoction) and 1 qian of Rhizoma Corydalis Yanhusuo (*Yuan Hu*). If there are no clots, the pain is a result of exposure to wind and cold. (In that case,) it is proper to administer ***Jia Jian Sheng Hua Tang*** (Modified Generating & Transforming Decoction).

Rhizoma Ligustici Wallichii (*Chuan Xiong*), 1 *qian*

Radix Angelicae Sinensis (*Dang Gui*), 4 *qian*
Rhizoma Carbonisata Zingiberis (*Hei Jiang*), 4 *fen*
Radix Praeparatus Glycyrrhizae (*Zhi Cao*), 4 *fen*
Radix Ledebouriellae Sesloidis (*Fang Feng*), 7 *fen*
Fructus Evodiae Rutecarpae (*Wu Yu*), 6 *fen*
Fructus Amomi Cardamomi (*Bai Dou Kou*), 5 *fen*
Ramulus Cinnamomi (*Gui Zhi*), 7 *fen*

After the pain is stopped, delete (what has been added). (Then) modify as instructed previously in accordance with the substance (or type of food which has caused) food injury.

Xiao Fu Tong
Lower Abdominal Pain

After delivery, the center is empty. If there is invasion of cold or drinking cold (drinks), cold may attack the lower abdomen giving rise to pain. (Such) pain can also be caused by blood clots or lumps, and, in addition, postpartum blood vacuity can result in pain below the navel. All (these types of pain) should be treated with ***Jia Jian Sheng Hua Tang*** (Modified Generating & Transforming Decoction).

Rhizoma Ligustici Wallichii (*Chuan Xiong*), 1 *qian*
Radix Angelicae Sinensis (*Dang Gui*), 3 *qian*
Rhizoma Carbonisata Zingiberis (*Hei Jiang*), 4 *fen*
Radix Praeparatus Glycyrrhizae (*Zhi Cao*), 4 *fen*
Semen Pruni Persicae (*Tao Ren*), 10 pieces

If there are lumps, this pain requires that this decoction (be administered) with *Qian Hu San* (Peucedanum Powder). Cold pain is also treated in the same way. Lower abdominal pain without clots and which can be relieved a little by pressure is (due to) blood vacuity. (For this,) add Radix Coquitus Rehmanniae (*Shu Di*), 3 *qian* and Radix Peucedani (*Qian Hu*) and

Cortex Cinnamomi (*Rou Gui*), each 1 *qian*, all powdered. (This is then) called *Qian Hu San*.

Xu Lao
Vacuity Taxation

The joints of the limbs are cold and painful with incessant sweating on the head.

Radix Panacis Ginseng (*Ren Shen*), 3 *qian*
Radix Angelicae Sinensis (*Dang Gui*), 3 *qian*
Radix Astragali Seu Hedysari (*Huang Qi*), 2 *qian*
Semen Praeparatus Sojae (*Dan Dou Chi*), 10 pieces
Rhizoma Recens Zingiberis (*Sheng Jiang*), 3 slices
Bulbus Allii Fistulosi (*Jiu Bai*), 10 *cun*
Pig's kidneys, 2

First, cook the kidneys well and then boil the medicinals in the soup down to 8/10. Take warm.

[A variant edition uses 1 pig's stomach instead of kidneys. This is boiled and then the medicinals are decocted in the soup.]

Bian Shen Teng Tong
Generalized Body Aching (&) Pain

During delivery the hundred joints open and extend and the blood vessels flow in a scattered way. With qi weak, the blood becomes retarded and stagnated around the channels and connecting vessels. If this does not disperse for days, then the sinews will contract, the vessels tug, and the bone joints will become inhibited. As a result, the lower and upper backs are unable to turn and the hands and feet are unable to move (even) the shoes. There may also be generalized fever and headache. If (this condition) is mistaken for cold injury and treated with effusion of the exterior through promoting perspiration, the sinews and vessels will become restless and the hands and feet will become cold, giving occasion to transmuted patterns. It is proper to administer ***Chen Tong San*** (Stifle Pain Powder).

Radix Angelicae Sinensis (*Dang Gui*), 1 *qian*
Radix Glycyrrhizae (*Gan Cao*)
Radix Astragali Seu Hedysari (*Huang Qi*)
Rhizoma Atractylodis Macrocephalae (*Bai Zhu*)
Radix Angelicae Duhuo (*Du Huo*), each 8 *fen*
Cortex Cinnamomi (*Rou Gui*), 8 *fen*
Ramus Loranthi Seu Visci (*Sang Ji Sheng*), 1 *qian*
Radix Achyranthis Bidentatae (*Niu Xi*), 8 *fen*
Bulbus Allii (*Xie Bai*), 5 pieces
Rhizoma Recens Zingiberis (*Jiang*), 3 slices

Decoct in water and take.

[In a variant edition there is no Ramus Loranthi Seu Visci.]

Yao Tong
Lumbar Pain

In women, the kidneys are tied to the uterus and the low back is the mansion of the kidneys. Therefore (low back pain) may be caused after delivery by taxation injury of the kidney qi, damage of the *bao luo* or connecting vessels of the uterus, or if wind assails before recovery from vacuity.

Yang Rong Zhuang Shen Tang (Nurture & Invigorate the Kidneys Decoction) [Treats postpartum invasion of wind cold and lumbar pain with inability to turn]

Radix Angelicae Sinensis (*Dang Gui*), 2 *qian*
Radix Ledebouriellae Sesloidis (*Fang Feng*), 4 *fen*
Radix Angelicae Duhuo (*Du Huo*)
Cortex Cinnamomi (*Gui Xin*)
Cortex Eucommiae Ulmoidis (*Du Zhong*)
Radix Dipsaci (*Xu Duan*)
Ramus Loranthi Seu Visci (*Sang Ji Sheng*), each 8 *fen*
Rhizoma Recens Zingiberis (*Sheng Jiang*), 3 slices

Decoct in water and take.

If, after 2 doses, the pain has not been relieved, the case is ascribed to kidney vacuity. (In that case, add Radix Coquitus Rehmanniae (*Shu Di*), 3 *qian*.

[In a variant edition there are 8 *fen* of Radix Ligustici Wallichii (*Chuan Xiong*).]

Jia Wei Da Zao Wan (Added Flavors Great Creation Pills) [Treat enduring postpartum dual vacuity of qi and blood with lumbar pain and weak kidneys. For their composition, see steaming bones (above).]

Qing E Wan (Young Beauty Pills)

Semen Juglandis Regiae (*Hu Tao*), 12 pieces
Fructus Psoraleae Corylifoliae (*Po Gu Zhi*), 8 *liang*, soaked in wine & stirred
Cortex Eucommiae Ulmoidis (*Du Zhong*), 1 *jin*, stir-fried with ginger juice, stripped of fiber

Powder fine and make into pills with heated honey. Take 60 pills with boiled, dilute vinegar (and) water.

[In a variant edition, Semen Juglandis Regiae is 20.]

Xie Tong
Lateral Costal Pain

(This is) due to blood vacuity and stagnant qi of the liver channel. In case of stagnant qi, prescribe *Si Jun Zi Tang* (Four Gentlemen Decoction) plus Pericarpium Viridis Citri Reticulatae (*Qing Pi*) and Radix Bupleuri (*Chai Hu*). In case of blood vacuity, prescribe *Si Wu Tang* (Four Ingredient Decoction) plus Radix Bupleuri, Radix Panacis Ginseng (*Ren Shen*), and Rhizoma Atractylodis Macrocephalae (*Bai Zhu*). Indiscriminate use of dry, aromatic medicinals will erroneously injure the clear and harmonious qi and (consequently) nothing can be generated.

Bu Fei San (Supplement the Lungs Powder) [Treats lateral costal pain]

Fructus Corni Officinalis (*Shan Yu*)
Radix Angelicae Sinensis (*Dang Gui*)
Fructus Schizandrae Chinensis (*Wu Wei*)
Radix Dioscoreae Oppositae (*Shan Yao*)
Radix Astragali Seu Hedysari (*Huang Qi*)
Rhizoma Ligustici Wallichii (*Chuan Xiong*)
Radix Coquitus Rehmanniae (*Shu Di*)
Fructus Chaenomelis Lagenariae (*Mu Gua*)
Rhizoma Atractylodis Macrocephalae (*Bai Zhu*)
Radix Angelicae Duhuo (*Du Huo*)
Semen Zizyphi Spinosae (*Zao Ren*), all in equal amounts

Decoct in water and take.

[In a variant edition, Fructus Corni Officinalis is 2 *qian*; Radix Angelicae Sinensis, 2 *qian*; Fructus Schizandrae Chinensis, 10 pieces; Radix Astragali Seu Hedysari, 8 *fen*; Rhizoma Ligustici Wallichii, 6 *fen*; Radix Coquitus Rehmanniae, 1.5 *qian*; Fructus

Chaenomelis Lagenariae and Rhizoma Atractylodis Macrocephalae, each 1 *qian*; Radix Angelicae Duhuo, 8 *fen*; Semen Zizyphi Spinosae, 1 *qian*; and Rhizoma Recens Zingiberis (*Jiang*), 1 slice. There is no Radix Dioscoreae Oppositae.]

Yin Tong
Genital Pain

If, after delivery, one begins to get around too soon, the birth gate may be invaded by wind thus causing such pain that the body dare not touch clothes or quilt. It is proper to use ***Qu Feng Ding Tong Tang*** (Dispel Wind & Settle Pain Decoction.)

Rhizoma Ligustici Wallichii (*Chuan Xiong*), 1 *qian*
Radix Angelicae Sinensis (*Dang Gui*), 3 *qian*
Radix Angelicae Duhuo (*Du Huo*)
Radix Ledebouriellae Sesloidis (*Fang Feng*)
Cortex Cinnamomi (*Rou Gui*)
Herba Seu Flos Schizonepetae Tenuifoliae (*Jing Jie*), char-fried, each 5 *fen*
Sclerotium Poriae Cocoris (*Fu Ling*), 1 *qian*
Radix Coquitus Rehmanniae (*Di Huang*), 2 *qian*
Fructus Zizyphi Jujubae (*Zao*), 2 pieces

Decoct and take.

Appendix on genital *gan* and genital erosion: Sores in the genitals are called private sores. They may be painful or itching like worms wriggling and from them dribbles a thick discharge. In nearly all the cases, genital erosion is due to stagnant qi and blood stasis due to vexed and depressed heart and kidneys and empty stomach qi. The classic states, "All types of sores with pain and itching are ascribed to the heart." The appropriate treatment is to supplement the heart and nurture the kidneys. Externally, one should fumigate and wash (the sore) with medicinals. It is proper to use ***Shi Quan Yin Gan San*** (All Ten Genital *Gan* Powder).

Rhizoma Ligustici Wallichii (*Chuan Xiong*)
Radix Angelicae Sinensis (*Dang Gui*)
Radix Albus Paeoniae Lactiflorae (*Bai Shao*)
Radix Sanguisorbae (*Di Yu*)
Radix Glycyrrhizae (*Gan Cao*), all in equal amounts

Boil in 5 bowls of water down to 2 bowls. Remove the dregs and then fumigate (the affected area) with the decoction 3 times in the day and 4 times at night. Fumigation should precede washing (also with this decoction).

Another method: Use 1 *sheng* of Pollen Typhae (*Pu Huang*) and 2 *liang* of mercury (*Shui Ying*). Mix and apply.

Another method: Use equal amounts of frog (*Xia Ma*) and rabbit droppings. Powder and apply to the sore.

Another method: Treats *gan* worms eating the lower part and the five viscera. Obtain a peach twig growing in the southeast part (of the tree). Lightly flail the end until frayed and then bandage (the sore) with the fibers.

Another method: Use powdered sulphur (*Shi Liu Huang*). Dab a frayed peach twig in the sulphur. Light it (on fire) in order to make smoke with which to fumigate (the affected area). [Note: It is necessary to combine this method with the one above.]

Another method: Take a short section of bamboo and insert it into the vagina. Then, burn a peach twig in order to produce smoke to fumigate (the vagina through this tube).

E Lou
The Lochia

This is the foul blood wrapping the child. If the lochia is discharged with delivery, there will be no abdominal pain and the delivery will go smoothly. (If) the abdomen is not warm enough or is injured by cold substances (*i.e.*, foods), the lochia will congeal into clots and be retained for a long time. This may give rise to a hundred emptiness conditions; (for instance,) possible generalized fever, steaming bone, low food intake and emaciation; or possibly vexatious heat in the five centers or menstrual stoppage. If the clots persist in the two flanks, there may occur thunderous rumbling on movement, a clamorous (stomach), dizziness, and malaria-like fever with fitful attacks. To treat these various conditions, one should first of all supplement vacuity if they want to drain the evil. To prevent the original qi from injury and to disperse the lochia, the only choice is to administer *Bu Zhong Yi Qi Tang* with *San Xiao Wan* (Three Dispersing Pills).

Jia Wei Bu Zhong Yi Qi Tang (Added Flavors Supplement the Center, Boost the Qi Decoction)

Radix Panacis Ginseng (*Ren Shen*), 1 *qian*
Rhizoma Atractylodis Macrocephalae (*Bai Zhu*), 2 *qian*
Radix Angelicae Sinensis (*Dang Gui*), 3 *qian*
Radix Praeparatus Astragali Seu Hedysari (*Huang Qi*), 1 *qian*
Radix Albus Paeoniae Lactiflorae (*Bai Shao*), 1 *qian*
Pericarpium Citri Reticulatae (*Guang Pi*), 4 *fen*
Radix Glycyrrhizae (*Gan Cao*), 4 *fen*
Rhizoma Recens Zingiberis (*Jiang*)
Fructus Zizyphi Jujubae (*Zao*)

Decoct and take.

San Xiao Wan (Three Dispersing Pills) [Treats the three conditions of dead blood, food accumulation, and phlegm in women]

Rhizoma Coptidis Chinensis (*Huang Lian*), 1 *liang*, half soaked & stir-fried in decocted Fructus Evodiae Rutecarpae (*Wu Yu*) with the dregs removed; half stir-fried in (decocted) Fructus Alpiniae Oxyphyllae (*Yi Zhi Ren*) which is discarded afterwards
Rhizoma Ligustici Wallichii (*Chuan Xiong*), 5 *qian*
Semen Raphani Sativi (*Lai Fu Zi*), 1 *liang* 5 *qian*, stir-fried
Semen Pruni Persicae (*Tao Ren*), 10 pieces
Fructus Gardeniae Jasminoidis (*Shan Zhi*)
Pericarpium Viridis Citri Reticulatae (*Qing Pi*)
Rhizoma Sparganii (*San Leng*)
Rhizoma Curcumae Zedoariae (*E Zhu*), each 5 *qian* & all stir-fried with vinegar
Fructus Crataegi (*Shan Zha*), 1 *liang*
Rhizoma Cyperi Rotundi (*Xiang Fu*), 1 *liang*, soaked & stir-fried in children's urine

Powder the above and make into pills after steaming in the form of a cake. Take between meals. Take 50-60 pills with *Bu Zhong Yi Qi Tang* or with 3 *qian* of Rhizoma Atractylodis Macrocephalae (*Bai Zhu*) and 5 *qian* of Pericarpium Citri Reticulatae (*Chen Pi*) which are boiled in 1 cup of water down to half.

[This formula treats postpartum food injury and retention of the lochia. For retention of lochia shortly after childbirth, it is proper to administer *Sheng Hua Tang* with 3 *qian* of charred Fructus Crataegi (*Shan Zha*) added. 1 dose per day. Best to take 4 *ji* in succession.]

Ru Yong
Mammary *Yong*

The nipples pertain to the foot *jue yin* liver channel. While the breasts pertain to the foot *yang ming* stomach channel. Swelling of the breasts with red nodules which several days afterwards become painful and rupture with sticky pus and then heal with the elimination of that pus is ascribed to toxic heat in the gallbladder with qi and blood stoppage and stagnation. (This is) called *ru* or mammary *yong* (and is) easy to cure. If, inside (the breast,) there develop small nodules which, initially, exhibit no red color and are not swollen or painful but last for years, growing larger and larger till they are like rugged, rocky mountains and (then) like ripe pomegranates when they break, (this is) difficult to cure. The treatment methods are to effuse the exterior to dissipate evils in case of pain, swelling, and alternating cold and hot; to course the liver and clear the stomach in case of severe pain; to expel from within in case of development of pus but refusal to rupture; to supplement the spleen and stomach in case of failing to grow (new) flesh with thin, clear pus; to supplement blood and qi in case of discharging pus and rupture with fever and aversion to cold; or to supplement the stomach qi in case of inability to eat or retching and vomiting. At the initial stage of *ru yan* or mammary rock, one should use *Yi Qi Yang Rong Tang* (Boost the Qi, Nurture Construction Decoction) with *Gui Pi Tang* (Return to the Spleen Decoction). Occasionally, it may be possible to disperse from within. (However,) the use of qi-moving and blood-cracking formulas only hastens death and that very rapidly.

Gua Lou San (Trichosanthis Powder) [Treats all types of *yong*, including mammary *yong*. *Yong* is (due to) disharmony of the qi of the six bowels. If yang stagnates within yin, (*yong*) may be generated.]

Fructus Trichosanthis Kirlowii (*Gua Lou*), 1 piece, unpeeled, smashed
Radix Glycyrrhizae (*Sheng Gan Cao*), 5 *fen*
Radix Angelicae Sinensis (*Dang Gui*), 3 *qian*
Gummum Olibani (*Ru Xiang*), 5 *fen*, stir-fried with Medulla Junci Effusi Tetrapanacis Papyriferi (*Deng Xin*)
Flos Lonicerae Japonicae (*Jin Yin Hua*), 3 *qian*
Radix Angelicae (*Bai Zhi*), 1 *qian*
Myrrha (*Mo Yao*), 5 *fen*, stir-fried with Medulla Tetrapancis Junci Effuse Papyriferi (*Deng Xin*)
Pericarpium Viridis Citri Reticulatae (*Qing Pi*), 5 *fen*

Decoct in water and take warm.

Hui Mai San (Recover the Pulse {or Vessels} Powder) [If taken before mammary *yong* ruptures, toxins are discharged through defecation. It should not be used in an empty person.]

Radix Et Rhizoma Rhei (*Da Huang*), 3.5 *qian*
Radix Angelicae (*Bai Zhi*), 8 *fen*
Gummum Olibani (*Ru Xiang*), 5 *fen*
Radix Saussureae Seu Vladimiriae (*Mu Xiang*), 5 *fen*
Myrrha (*Mo Yao*), 5 *fen*
Squama Manitis (*Chuan Shan Jia*), 5 *fen*, mixed & fried with powdered clam shell

Grind into powder. Decoct 2 *qian* of Radix Panacis Ginseng (*Ren Shen*), mix in the powdered medicinals, and take.

[In a variant edition Radix Et Rhizoma Rhei is 3 *qian* and there are also 3 *qian* of Radix Panacis Ginseng.]

Shi Quan Da Bu Tang (Ten Complete Great Supplementing Decoction)

Radix Panacis Ginseng (*Ren Shen*)
Rhizoma Atractylodis Macrocephalae (*Bai Zhu*)
Radix Astragali Seu Hedysari (*Huang Qi*)
Radix Coquitus Rehmanniae (*Shu Di*), each 3 *qian*
Sclerotium Poriae Cocoris (*Fu Ling*), 8 *fen*
Radix Glycyrrhizae (*Gan Cao*), 5 *fen*
Rhizoma Ligustici Wallichii (*Chuan Xiong*), 8 *fen*
Flos Lonicerae Japonicae (*Jin Yin Hua*), 3 *qian*

In case of diarrhea, add Rhizoma Coptidis Chinensis (*Huang Lian*) and Semen Myristicae Fragrantis (*Rou Guo*). In case of thirst, add Tuber Ophiopogonis Japonicae (*Mai Dong*) and Fructus Schizandrae Chinensis (*Wu Wei*). In case of alternating fever and chills, use pounded *Ma Ti Xiang*.[7] For any type of mammary *yong*, it is beneficial to administer Semen Coicis Lachryma-jobi (*Yi Yi Ren*) gruel. Another formula: 5 *qian* of Radix Linderae Strychnifoliae (*Wu Yao*) and softened, hot *Bai Xiang*,[8] ground and boiled with 1 slice of ox-hide gelatin (*Niu Pi Jiao*) in 1 bowl of water down to 7/10. Take warm. For abdominal *yong* in pregnant women, either of these two formulas may be used.

[In a variant edition Radix Panacis Ginseng and the other three ingredients are each 2 *qian*.]

In addition, *ru chui* or blown breast, which is caused by the blowing of the baby's mouth qi when sucking milk, is the stoppage of milk due to congestion and binding. If not treated immediately, this will develop into *yong*. It is, (therefore,)

7 Identification not clear. Either Lignum Aquillariae Agallochae or Radix Asari Forbesii. Both are sometimes referred to as *Ma Ti Xiang*.

8 Identification not clear. Either Lignum Aquilariae Agallochae or Radix Saussaureae Seu Vladimiriae (*Bai Mu Xiang*).

appropriate to administer *Gua Lou San* without delay and to also rub (the breast) with the hand to dissipate (the congestion).

Feng Shen
Severe Wind

Collect fresh goat's blood, bake it dry on a new clay tile, and grind it. Take 5-6 *fen* per dose mixed with old wine. In serious cases, use as much as 8 *fen*. It is miraculously effective.

Another (method): Bake till dry on a clay tile an aborted chicken egg. Mix with wine and take.

For the treatment of critical conditions of empty cold, use the root bark of *Lan Xu Zi*[9], bake till dry on a new tile, and grind. Take warm, 1 *qian* per dose. No matter how dangerous, 1,000 (cases) are completely guaranteed.

Bu Yu
Aphasia

Due to malign blood stagnating and accumulating in the heart, heart qi is blocked and the tongue becomes rigid with loss of speech. Use ***Qi Zhen San*** (Seven Pearls Powder).

Radix Panacis Ginseng (*Ren Shen*)
Rhizoma Acori Graminei (*Shi Chang Pu*)
Rhizoma Ligustici Wallichii (*Chuan Xiong*)
Radix Rehmanniae (*Sheng Di*), each 1 *qian*
Cinnabaris (*Chen Sha*), 5 *fen*, ground

---

9 Unidentifiable; possibly Radix Isatidis Seu Baphicacanthi (*Ban Lan Geng*)

Radix Ledebouriellae Sesloidis (*Fang Feng*), 5 *qian*
Herba Cum Radice Asari Sieboldi (*Xi Xin*), 1 *qian*

Grind into a fine powder. Use *Bo He Tang* (Mint Decoction) (to chase) down 1 *qian*. (For) speechlessness due to depression and binding of phlegm qi, use 1 *qian* of good quality Alum (*Ming Fan*) ground with water. (Chase) down with boiling water.

Another formula to treat postpartum loss of speech:

Radix Panacis Ginseng (*Ren Shen*)
Semen Nelumbinis Nuciferae (*Shi Lian Zi*), cored
Rhizoma Acori Graminei (*Shi Chang Pu*), all in equal amounts

Decoct in water and take.

The *Fu Ren Liang Fang* says:

> (In terms of) postpartum loss of voice, inability to utter owing to vacuity of the heart and kidneys (requires) *Qi Zhen San*; depression and binding of spleen qi (requires) *Gui Pi Tang* (Return to the Spleen Decoction); spleen injury (due to) low food (intake requires) *Si Jun Zi Tang* (Four Gentlemen Decoction); dual vacuity of qi and blood (requires) *Ba Zhen Tang* (Eight Pearls Decoction) (or), in case of failure to respond, *Du Shen Tang* (Solitary Ginseng Decoction). It is particularly inappropriate to add Radix Praeparatus Aconiti Carmichaeli (*Fu Zi*) impetuously, since blood is generated through supplementing the blood. If one only uses *Fu Shou San* (Buddha's Hand Powder)[10] or other such blood-cracking medicinals, this is a serious mistake.

---

10 This is composed of equal amounts of Radix Angelicae Sinensis (*Dang Gui*) and Rhizoma Ligustici Wallichii (*Chuan Xiong*) in large amounts.

Bu Bian
Appendix

Chan Hou Da Bian Bu Tong
Postpartum Constipation

Use *Sheng Hua Tang* with Semen Cannabis Sativae (*Ma Ren*) instead of Rhizoma Carbonisata Zingiberis (*Hei Jiang*). In case of fullness and distention, add Pericarpium Citri Reticulatae (*Chen Pi*). In case of blood clot pain, add Cortex Cinnamomi (*Rou Gui*) and Rhizoma Corydalis Yanhusuo (*Yan Hu*). If dryness and binding have lasted more than ten days, there must be dry feces in the anus. (Therefore,) use a honey jujube (*i.e.*, a date-like suppository) to conduct.

Processing Method for Honey Dates

(Take) good honey, 2-3 *liang*. Heat it to boiling and do not stop till it turns to a tea-brown color. Pour onto a moistened table and shape by hand into a jujuba (or date-like suppository). Put this into the anus and retain till a desire appears to defecate. Remove the honey date and defecate.

Another method: Hold sesame oil in the mouth, insert a bamboo tube into the anus, and then blow in 4-5 mouthfuls of oil. When (the oil) has mixed with the feces in the intestine, the bowels will relax. Pig bile can be used as a substitute.

Zhi Chan Hou Ji Zhao Feng
Treating Postpartum Chicken Claw Wind

Lignum Carbonisatum Mori Albi (*Sang Chai Hui*), 3 *qian*, with nature preserved
Fish gelatin (*Yu Jiao*), 3 *qian*, stir-fried
Human nail, 12 pieces, stir-fried

Grind into powder and take with Shaoxing wine. When there is sweat, the cure is affected.

Bao Chan Wu San (Worry-free Childbirth-protecting Powder)

Radix Angelicae Sinensis (*Dang Gui*), 1.5 *qian*, washed with wine
Herba Seu Flos Carbonisatus Schizonepetae Tenuifoliae (*Chao Hei Jie Sui*), 8 *fen*
Rhizoma Ligustici Wallichii (*Chuan Xiong*), 1.5 *qian*
Folium Artemesiae Argyii (*Ai Ye*), 7 *fen*, stir-fried
Fructus Praeparatus Citri Seu Ponciri (*Mian Chao Zhi Qiao*), 6 *fen*
Radix Praeparatus Astragali Seu Hedysari (*Zhi Huang Qi*), 8 *fen*
Semen Cuscutae (*Tu Si Zi*), 1.4 *qian*, stir-fried with wine
Cortex Magnoliae Officinalis (*Hou Po*), 7 *fen*, stir-fried with ginger
Radix Et Rhizoma Notopterygii (*Qiang Huo*), 5 *fen*
Bulbus Fritillariae Cirrhosae (*Chuan Bei Mu*), 1 *qian*, cored
Radix Albus Paeoniae Lactiflorae (*Bai Shao*), 1.2 *qian*, stir-fried with wine
Radix Glycyrrhizae (*Gan Cao*), 5 *fen*
Rhizoma Recens Zingiberis (*Jiang*), 3 slices

Take warm.

The above formula protects the fetus. Take 3-5 times per month. Towards delivery, take warm. Hastens delivery in a miraculous way.

Zhi Pian Ti Fu Zhong Treating Generalized Water Swelling

(This is) caused by water spillage due to spleen vacuity. (The following) is applicable to any type of water swelling (and is) always miraculously effective.

Fructus Seu Semen Amomi (*Zhen Suo Sha Ren*), 4 *liang*
Semen Raphani Sativi·(*Lai Fu Zi*), 2 *liang*, 4 *qian*

Grind and dip (the Semen Raphani Sativi) in water. Extract from it the juice when it is fully soaked. Soak the Fructus Seu Semen Amomi in this till all the juice has been absorbed. Then dry the Fructus Seu Semen Amomi in the sun and finally grind it very fine. Take 1 qian at a time, gradually increasing the dosage to 2 qian at the most. Take with dilute, boiled ginger water.

Bao Chan Shen Xiao Fang (Divinely Effective Childbirth-protecting Formula)

(This formula) is able to ensure safety before delivery and to hasten delivery during labor. In case of accidentally injured fetal qi with lumbar and abdominal pain or even in case of incessant bleeding bordering on abortion — a critical situation — take once for a cure; take twice (and) everything (will be) calm. In case of failure of the joined bones to move in the course of labor, transverse or inverted presentation, or death within the abdomen with (the mother's) life at stake, take it and a magical effect will be wrought.

Radix Angelicae Sinensis (*Quan Dang Gui*), 1.5 *qian*, washed with wine
Cortex Magnoliae Officinalis (*Zi Hou Po*), 7 *fen*, stir-fried with ginger juice
Rhizoma Ligustici Wallichii (*Zhen Chuan Xiong*), 1.5 *qian*
Semen Cuscutae (*Tu Si Zi*), 1.5 *qian*, soaked with wine
Bulbus Fritillariae Cirrhosae (*Chuan Bei Mu*), 2 *qian*, cored, boiled separately, & added afterwards
Fructus Citri Seu Ponciri (*Zhi Qiao*), 6 *fen*, stir-fried with flour
Radix Et Rhizoma Notopterygii (*Chuan Qiang Huo*), 6 *fen*
Herba Seu Flos Schizonepetae Tenuifoliae (*Jing Jie Sui*), 8 *fen*
Radix Astragali Seu Hedysari (*Huang Qi*), 8 *fen*, fried with honey
Folium Artemesiae Argyii (*Qi Ai*), 5 *fen*, stir-fried with vinegar
Radix Praeparatus Glycyrrhizae (*Zhi Cao*), 5 *fen*
Radix Albus Paeoniae Lactiflorae (*Bai Shao*), 1.2 *qian*, 2 *qian* in winter, stir-fried with wine
Rhizoma Recens Zingiberis (*Jiang*), 3 slices

Boil in 2 bowls of water down to 8/10. (Then) boil 1 cup of the decoction with the dregs down to 6/10. Towards but before delivery, take 2 *ji* on an empty stomach. During labor, take it warm at any time.

[Note: Worry-free Childbirth-protecting Powder and the Divinely Effective Childbirth-protecting Formulas are the same as the Secret Proven Efficacious Formula for the treatment of parturient cases given in the beginning section; only the explanations are a little different. These can be cross-referenced.]

Index

A

abdominal aching 43, 45, 66, 117
abdominal pain 10, 41-45, 48, 66, 69, 73, 75, 78, 87-91, 93, 117, 118, 144, 147, 159, 160, 212, 214, 216, 227, 232, 237, 238, 239, 246, 255
abnormal position 97
abortion 66, 69, 70, 73, 74, 78, 80, 81, 87, 89, 90, 161, 255
aching & pain below the umbilicus 47
acid regurgitation 24, 129
acupuncture 112
agitation 78, 79, 86, 105, 107, 203
alternating cold and heat 129
alternating fever and chills 40, 41, 47, 142, 187, 188, 191, 250
amenorrhea 22, 55
An Dian Er Tian Tang 66
An Lao Tang 39
An Shen Ding Zhi Wan 180
An Shen Sheng Hua Tang 180
An Shen Wan 144
An Xin Tang 113
ancient formulas 163, 167
anger 13, 80, 90, 132, 174, 184-186
angry depression 186
angry qi 81, 177, 186
anterior secret organ 53
aphasia 251
aversion to cold 88, 122, 160, 187, 190, 223, 229, 248
aversion to wind and cold 200

B

Ba Wei Di Huang Wan 201
Ba Zhen Tang 147, 149, 204, 229, 252
baby gate 95
baby's mouth qi 250
bai dai 4, 5
balancing (or regulating) delivery 148
balancing the menses 31, 46, 48
Bao Chan Shen Xiao Fang 255
bao gong 3, 23
bao luo 241
bao tai 3, 8, 23, 28, 47, 52, 53, 66, 69, 70, 72, 90, 94, 101, 107, 125, 127, 131
bao tai ligation 52, 66, 90
Bao He Tang 252
Bao Zhen Tang 235
beng lou 20, 22
bian shen teng tong 240
bian shu 209
birth gate 93, 95, 99, 101, 102, 127, 131, 133, 143, 244
birthing & afterwards 207
black vaginal discharge 10, 11
blood accumulation 25
blood chamber 21, 41, 47, 48, 85, 109, 111, 113, 118
blood clots 38, 42, 142, 163, 183, 199, 200, 219, 230, 233, 239
blood dizziness 105, 109, 162, 166, 168, 170, 182
blood lump pain 170, 171, 182
blood lumps 157, 164, 178, 185, 237
blood vessels 23, 24, 240
blown breast 250

body heat 160, 165, 177, 191, 224
bone marrow 26, 33
breach presentation 97
breast distention 136
breast milk 134-136, 154
bright red blood 175
bright, shiny skin complexion 226
broken uterus 127, 128
bu an 66, 85
Bu Fei San 243
bu gu 3, 51, 85
Bu Pao Yin 207
Bu Qi Jie Yun Tang 110
Bu Qi Yang Rong Tang 178
Bu Qin Sheng Chang Yin 115
Bu Xue Tang 20, 54, 65, 111

bu yu 111, 251
Bu Zhong Yi Qi Tang 64, 65, 108, 143, 180, 182, 217, 226, 229, 231, 246, 247

C

central qi 126, 162, 193, 230
Chai Hu Mei Lian Tang 235
Chai Hu Tang 190, 223
chan hou 117, 120, 122, 123, 125, 127, 131, 132, 134, 135, 139, 141, 157, 159, 163, 205, 207, 253, 254
chan hou e han shen chan 122
chan hou e xin ou tu 123
chan hou gan wei 132
chan hou han re 159
chan hou qi chuan 120
chan hou qi xue liang xu ru ye bu xia 134
chan hou rou xian chu 131
chan hou shao fu tong 117
chan hou shou shang bao tai lin li bu zhi 127
chan hou xue beng 125
chan hou yong yao shi wu 157
chan hou yu jie ru ye bu tong 135
chan men 95, 101
Chang Ning Tang 119
Chang Sheng Huo Ming Dan 143
Chen Tong San 241
Chen Zi-ming 193
Cheng Qi Tang 165, 192
chi dai 12, 14
child dead at the birth gate 101
child's pillow pain 117
choleric diseases 219
chong and *ren* 9, 47, 48
chong mai 28, 47
chronic afflictions 24
chu han 198
cinnabar 8
Classic of Change 12
clouding 18, 19, 85, 86, 105, 107, 111, 125, 149, 164, 166, 167
clouding and dizziness 105, 111, 125, 149, 164
cold coughing 176, 177
cold diarrhea 210, 212, 214
cold feet 178
cold injury before delivery 161
complexion desertion 168, 169, 199, 212
conception 3, 8, 23, 48, 53, 57, 61, 131, 132
conception vessel 8, 9, 48
confused speech 179
confused vision and hearing 173
Cong Yun Fa 228
connecting vessels of the uterus 227, 241
constipation 86, 159, 162, 176, 179, 192, 193, 195, 226, 230, 232, 238, 253
constructive qi 4
consummate yin 13, 55
consumption pattern 46
contusion 3, 21, 26, 27, 73, 74, 85
convulsions 197
cool injury 143
copious sweating 194, 196, 199-201, 203
counterflow chilling 171, 220, 229
counterflow retching (&) inability to eat 221
cracked lips 86
crying from within the abdomen 77
cui sheng 149, 155
Cui Sheng Tu Nao Wan 155
cun kou pulses 19

D

da beng 76
da bian gan jie xiao chan 86
da nu xiao chan 90
dai bing 4
dai mai 3, 6, 8, 13, 66, 131, 132
dai xia 3, 4, 8
Dan-xi 141, 145, 190
Dang Gui Bu Xue Tang 20, 65, 111
Dang Gui Liu Huang Tang 199, 202
dao han 199, 201
dark eyes 18, 109
dark purple blood clots 42
dead child within the abdomen 102
defecation 162, 215, 217, 231, 249
defensive qi 4
delayed menstruation 34
depression 7, 13, 24-26, 35-38, 41-43, 54-57, 71-73, 135, 136, 141, 144, 186,

230, 252
depression knotting profuse bleeding 24
desertion of blood 166
desire to retch 123, 125
desire to run 113
desire to vomit 109
diarrhea 69, 71, 166, 171, 193, 210-218, 220, 250
die shan xiao chan 85
difficult delivery 93, 95, 97, 99, 101-103, 128, 148, 149, 151, 153
diffuse swellings 228
diminished food intake 166
Ding Jing Tang 36
distressed, rapid breathing 157
dizziness 17, 18, 105, 107, 109-112, 125, 126, 145, 149, 162, 164, 166-170, 173, 182, 222, 246
dong chan 149
dragon-thunderous fire 80
dry mouth 24, 67, 192, 194
dry mouth & sore throat in pregnancy 67
dry throat 203
dry, bound stools 142, 194, 230
du 3, 21, 28, 38, 54, 57, 67, 70, 86, 126, 132, 148, 154, 169, 171, 241-244, 252
Du Huo Tang 148
duan qi 153
Duo Ming Dan 156
duo tai 80, 90, 161
dysentery 213, 215-219
dyspnea 120, 121, 129, 165, 180, 181, 200, 227

E

e lou 246
e xue 160
earlier heaven 66, 89
earlier heaven true fire 89
earlier heaven true qi 89
early menstruation 31, 32
emaciation 54, 246
enuresis 132, 204, 209
epidemic disease 161, 162
er men 95, 114
er zhen zhi teng 117
essence 4, 8, 20, 22-24, 29, 34, 36, 38, 45, 49, 54-57, 61, 64, 66, 68, 69, 73, 80, 83, 84, 87, 88, 93, 96, 121, 125, 126, 128, 130, 182, 194, 199
essence chamber 29
essence spirit 54, 55, 128, 194
evil spirit 180
excessive menstruation 49
exhaustion 4, 142, 166, 194
external injury 27, 73, 74
external invasion 36, 37, 40, 142, 160, 190, 194, 223-225
external invasion of wind cold 40, 223-225
external treatment 30, 127, 164-167
extraordinary transmuted patterns 99, 115

F

faintness 85, 86
falling fetus 80, 90
fatigue 49, 61, 141, 149, 165, 166, 168, 171, 177, 192, 199, 203, 213, 228, 229, 233
fatigue arising on movement 229
fatigued limbs 63
fecal stoppage 154, 196
fei fen 160
fen nu 184
feng shen 251
fetal crying in pregnancy 77
fetal death 151, 154
fetal disorders 64
fetal education 22
fetal heat 77
fetal leakage 75
fetal mania 78
fetal suspension 71-73
fetus 3, 22, 23, 28, 61, 64, 66-75, 77-82, 85, 87, 89, 90, 93, 94, 97, 100, 104, 106, 109, 113, 117, 147, 148, 150-152, 154, 155, 156, 159, 255
fever 40, 41, 47, 113, 122, 129, 142, 160, 162, 165, 187, 188, 190, 191, 192, 194, 224, 236, 240, 246, 248, 250
fire qi 32, 78, 79, 87, 89, 121

five viscera 34, 78, 88, 93, 245
flowery vision 109, 166
fluid collapse 201
food accumulation 37, 141, 210, 215, 247
food injury 66, 141, 171, 176, 177, 179, 182, 184, 186, 194, 217, 218, 230, 231, 238, 239, 247
foot *jue yin* liver channel 248
foot *yang ming* stomach channel 248
form desertion 162, 170, 173, 174, 211
frequent diarrhea 216
frequent urination 209, 229
fright 141, 143, 149, 174, 176, 197, 198, 233, 237
fright palpitations 143, 197, 233, 237
fright palpitations with restlessness 237
frozen delivery 149
fu ke 193
Fu Qi Zhi Ti Tang 77
Fu Ren Liang Fang 193, 252
Fu Ren Liang Fang Da Quan 193
Fu Shen Tang 172, 177, 181, 182
Fu Shou San 252
fu tong 117, 238, 239
Fu Zi San 220
fullness in the center 230

G

gallbladder 235, 248
gan fen 160
gan wei 132
gan worms 245
generalized fatigue 49, 229
generalized fever 160, 165, 191, 224, 240, 246
generalized water swelling 255
genital erosion 244
genital *gan* 244, 245
genital pain 244
gestational diseases 82
girdle vessel 3, 13
green-blue vaginal discharge 6, 7
Gu Ben Zhi Beng Tang 17
gu fang 167
Gu Qi Tang 21
Gu Qi Tian Jing Tang 83
gu zheng 235
Gua Lou San 248, 251
Gui Pi Tang 234, 248, 252
gynecology 1, 59, 193

H

hastening birth 100, 104, 149
he gan 15
He Gu 98
headache 149, 187, 188, 190, 191, 194, 224, 240
heart 11, 13, 52-57, 66, 70, 71, 78, 79, 85, 90, 105, 109-115, 125, 143, 148, 149, 164, 167, 174, 182, 198, 222, 233, 234, 237, 244, 251, 252
heart pain 237
heat inside the bones 33
heavenly cold 149
heavy voice 223, 224
hei dai 10
hemafecia prior to menstruation 52
hematuria during pregnancy 75
heng chan 150
hesitation in movement 113
honey jujube 253
hot delivery 149
hot diarrhea 210, 212
hou tian 66
hou tian spleen 66
Hua Tai San 154
huang dai 4, 8, 9
Huang Di Nei Jing 145
Hui Mai San 249
human reproductive function 38
hun 17, 19, 109, 179
huo luan 219
hypertonicity of the sinews 195

I

ill-practiced midwife 207
impact injury in pregnancy 73
imperial and ministerial fires 28
incessant sweating 199, 240
incessant sweating on the head 240
incessant vomiting 220
incontinence of defecation 217
indignation (&) anger 184

inflation (&) distention 230
inhibited urination 165, 203
injured delivery 147, 148
injured fetal origin 73
insufficient food intake 229
interior vexation 222
internal injury 27, 36, 37, 45, 73
interstices 40
inversion condition 171

J

ji ji diagram 12
ji ji way 31, 52
Ji Kun Dan 159
Jia Jian Bu Zhong Yi Qi Tang 64
Jia Jian Dang Gui Bu Xue Tang 20
Jia Jian Sheng Hua Tang 198, 211, 216, 221, 238, 239
Jia Jian Si Wu Tang 50, 88
Jia Jian Xiao Yao San 7
Jia Jian Yang Rong Tang 233
Jia Jian Yang Wei Tang 188
Jia Shen An Fei Sheng Hua Tang 224
Jia Shen Sheng Hua Tang 143, 145, 164, 169-172, 178, 180, 182, 199, 230
Jia Wei Bu Zhong Yi Qi (Tang) 199
Jia Wei Da Zao Wan 236, 242
Jia Wei Sheng Hua Tang 114, 125, 166, 168, 183, 191, 213, 223, 238
Jia Wei Si Wu Tang 41, 225
Jia Wei Xiong Gui Tang 151
Jian Gu Tang 51
Jian Pi Hua Shi San Qi Tang 186
Jian Pi Li Shui Sheng Hua Tang 211
Jian Pi Tang 231
Jian Pi Xiao Shi Sheng Hua Tang 183
Jiang Zi Tang 96, 97
jiao gan xue chu 22
jiao gu bu kai nan chan 95
jiao shou xian xia nan chan 97
Jie Yu Tang 72
jin ye 201
jing bi 22, 56
jing essence 8, 22, 23, 61
jing ji 233
jing qian da bian xia xue 52
jing qian xie shui 51
jing shen 54, 128
jing shui 4, 31, 33, 35, 37, 38, 40, 42, 47, 49, 55
jing shui guo duo 49
jing shui hou qi 33
jing shui jiang lai qi xia xian teng tong 47
jing shui wei lai fu xian teng 42
jing shui xian hou wu ding qi 35
jing shui xian qi 31
Jing Yue Quan Shu 202
Jiu Bai Qiu Sheng Tang 125
Jiu Mu Dan 101
Jiu Sun An Tai Tang 74
joined bones 95, 96, 99-101, 151, 255

K

ke sou 223
kidney fire 9, 123, 129
kidney water 39, 43, 55, 56, 61, 68, 72, 78, 83, 123, 129
kidneys 8, 9, 13, 31, 32, 34-36, 38, 44-46, 52-57, 61, 63, 66, 69, 70-73, 87, 90, 93, 121, 123-125, 129, 130, 226, 240, 241, 242, 244, 252
knotted lumps 164, 228
kou ke jian xiao bian bu li 203

L

lactation 135, 179
languor 49
lao nian jing shui fu xing 38
lao nian xue beng 19
lao wei nian jing shui duan 55
lao zheng 46
large intestine 52-54, 87, 119
late periods 33, 34
lateral costal pain 129, 142, 190, 223, 243
latter heaven 66
lei jing 197
lei nue 187
lei shang han 190, 192
lei zhong feng 195
li 11, 40, 80, 85, 98, 106, 127, 168, 176, 189, 196, 200, 202, 203, 209, 211, 213, 215, 224, 226, 234
LI 4 98

Li Huo Tang 11
Li Qi San Yu Tang 85
Li Qi Xie Huo Tang 80
Liang Di Tang 33
Liang Shou Tang 131
Liao Er San 103
life gate 10, 13
life mechanism 103
lin 13, 127, 208
Liu Qi Yin Zi 185
liu zhu 228
liver 4-7, 13-15, 24, 25, 28, 29, 34-46, 53-57, 61-63, 72, 73, 80, 81, 90, 91, 109, 121, 129, 130, 132-134, 136, 160, 174, 186, 188, 198, 243, 248
liver atony 132
liver phase 160
lochia 113, 114, 125, 142, 144, 158, 210, 216, 227, 228, 230, 231, 246, 247
loss of consciousness 17, 166, 211
loss of speech 111, 251, 252
lower abdominal pain 43, 66, 117, 118, 239
lower abdominal pain in pregnancy 66
lower back 13
lower burner 8, 47
lower orifice 4
lumbar pain 194, 241, 242
lump pain 144, 158, 168, 170-173, 180-182, 184, 191, 199, 220, 232, 238
lump stuck in the throat 56
lung phase 160
lungs 64, 65, 69, 120, 203, 224, 243

M

Ma Er Huang Liu San 143
Ma Huang Geng Tang 200
Ma Huang Tang 190, 223
maidens 4
malaria 142, 161, 187-189, 246
malign blood 26, 109, 125, 160, 164, 167, 251
malign toxin 127
mammary rock 248
mammary *yong* 248-250
mania 41, 78, 79, 112-114
mania in pregnancy 78
mania-like disease 41
married women 4
menstrual block 22, 55-57
menstrual counterflow 45, 46
menstrual flow 4, 23, 29, 33-36, 38, 40, 42, 43, 47, 49-53, 55, 56, 68
menstruation ahead of schedule 31
menstruation behind schedule 33
midwife 127, 128, 148, 150, 207
ming men 10, 13, 38
ming men zhi huo 38
ministerial fire 80
miscarriage 21, 69, 83-88, 90, 154, 157, 161
miscarriage (due to) great anger 90
miscarriage (due to) wrenching & contusion 85
miscarriage with dry, knotted stools 86
miscellaneous disease 210
morning sickness 61-63
Mu Xiang Bing Lang Wan 185
Mu Xiang Sheng Hua Tang 185

N

nan chan 93, 95, 97, 99, 101, 102, 151
nasal congestion 223
navel 13, 25, 41, 48, 80, 153, 218, 239
needling 98, 112
Nei Jing 55, 145
nei shang 36
new blood 26, 85, 106, 109, 142, 159, 195
ni zheng 171
night sweating 199, 202
normal delivery 105, 109, 111, 112, 114, 147
normal delivery (but) intestinal prolapse 114
nu ke 1, 59
nuns 4

O

old blood 26, 106, 109
onion-ironing method 228
oppression 71, 73, 87, 144, 158, 183, 184, 230
origin evils 8

original qi 12, 35, 154, 184, 187, 212, 215, 217, 246
ou ni bu shi 221
overeating 148, 183, 210, 213, 230
oversleep 148

P

pain in the breasts 136
pain in the lumbar region 77
pain in their lateral costal regions 71
pan chang chan 150, 151
parched tongue 67
pedicle of the placenta 105
penetrating vessel 28, 48
peng zhang 230
pericardium 113
periumbilical pain 148
pian ti fu zhong 255
ping gan 15, 25
Ping Wei San 152, 153
placenta 3, 95, 102, 105-108, 147, 149, 150, 152, 153, 159, 189
po 27, 104, 153, 155, 158, 165, 179, 207, 216, 218, 220, 226, 227, 242, 254, 256
portals 24, 76, 114, 135
postpartum anger 184
postpartum asthma 120
postpartum aversion to cold 122, 160
postpartum cold (&) heat 159
postpartum dizziness 169, 173, 182
postpartum enduring dysentery 218, 219
postpartum exit of fleshy fiber 131
postpartum heart and abdominal pain 237
postpartum incessant dribbling 127
postpartum injury (due to) cold 122
postpartum liver atony 132
postpartum lower abdominal pain 117, 118
postpartum nausea, retching, (&) vomiting 123
postpartum profuse (uterine) bleeding 125
postpartum vexation 203
postpartum windstroke 231
pregnancy 21, 22, 31, 48, 61, 63, 64, 66, 67, 69, 71, 73-75, 77, 78, 79-81, 84, 87, 89, 96, 144, 214
pregnancy malign blockage 61
premature menopause 55, 56
private sores 244
profuse (uterine) bleeding 17, 22, 24, 38, 40, 69, 84, 125, 126, 145, 174
profuse bleeding due to wrenching & falling 26
profuse bleeding in old women 19
profuse bleeding in young women 21
profuse sweating 165, 170, 173-176, 179, 197, 201, 204, 222, 224
Pu Xiao Jian 152
pulse desertion 170
pus 229, 230, 248

Q

qi barrier 107
qi counterflow difficult delivery 99
qi desertion 83, 85, 168, 181, 182
qi duan si chuan 177
qi exhaustion 166
qi guan 107
qi ni nan chan 99
Qi Zhen San 251, 252
Qian Hu San 239
Qiang Huo Yang Rong Tang 143
qing dai 6
Qing E Wan 242
Qing Gan Zhi Lin Tang 13
Qing Gu San 235, 236
Qing Hai Wan 29
Qing Jing San 32
Qing Xue Wan 217
Qu Feng Ding Tong Tang 244
quasi-cold injury 171, 190, 192, 193
quasi-malaria 187, 188
quasi-*shao yang* pattern 190
quasi-*tai yang* pattern 190
quasi-tetany 197
quasi-windstroke 195

R

racing heart 233
re chan 149

rectal heaviness 215, 216, 218
recurrent menstruation in old women 38
red facial complexion 10, 149, 223
red vaginal discharge 12-14
reddish yellow, watery stools 210
ren mai 8, 9, 47
ren shen die sun 73
ren shen e zu 61
ren shen fu zhong 63
ren shen guo nu duo tai 80
ren shen kou gan yan teng 67
ren shen shao fu teng 66
ren shen tu xie fu teng 69
ren shen xiao bian xia xue 75
ren shen yao fu teng 78
ren shen zi ming 77
ren shen zi xuan xie teng 71
restless fetus 68
restless stirring of the fetus 66
retching 24, 25, 27, 61, 62, 109, 123, 124, 221, 222, 229, 248
retention of blood clots 200
retention of lochia 113, 142, 247
righteous and evil fire 42
rigid cold 187
ru chui 250
ru yan 248
ru yong 248
rubbing and pressing 184
Run Chang Zhou 195
Run Zao An Tai Tang 68

S

San Jie Ding Tong Tang 118
San Xiao Wan 246
Sang Piao San 209
sea of blood 28-30, 47, 48, 51
sea of water and grain 78
secret gate 4, 10
severe fatigue 165, 166, 168, 177, 199
severe wind 251
severing the navel 153
severing the umbilical cord 153
sexual affairs 37
sexual desire 20, 22, 24, 84
sexual intercourse 3, 19, 21-24, 28, 29, 66, 83, 84, 96, 125, 127
sexual qi 23
(sexual) union causing bleeding 22
shan die xue beng 26
Shan Zha Tang 159
shang chan 147, 148
shang liang 143
shang shi 182
shang tai yuan 73
shao fu xue beng 21
shao yang pattern 190
shao yin condition 192
Shen Gui Sheng Hua Tang 228
Shen Ling Sheng Hua Tang 214
Shen Xian Hui Dong San 229
Shen Zhu Gao 189
Sheng Hua Liu He Tang 219
Sheng Hua Tang 114, 125, 142-145, 152, 157-160, 162-175, 178, 180, 182-187, 191, 195, 198, 199, 210, 211, 213-218, 221, 223, 224, 228, 230, 232, 233, 237, 238, 239, 247, 253
sheng ji 103
Sheng Jin Yi Ye Tang 222
Sheng Jin Zhi Ke Yi Shui Yin 203
Sheng Ju Da Bu Tang 174, 175, 177, 182
Sheng Mai San 162, 171, 204
Sheng Ru Dan 135
Sheng Xue Zhi Beng Tang 175
Shi Lian San 222
Shi Quan Da Bu Tang 122, 249
Shi Quan Da Bu Wan 229
Shi Quan Yin Gan San 245
Shi Xiao San 152, 153, 238
shivering 122
shortness of breath similar to asthma 177
Shou Mo Tang 133
shu gan 15
Shu Qi San 100
shui gu li 213
shui gu zhi hai 78
shui zhong 218, 226
Shun Jing Liang An Tang 53

si chan 101, 151
Si Jun Zi Tang 243, 252
Si Ni Tang 171
Si Wu Tang 41, 50, 62, 63, 88, 157, 218, 225, 229, 243
Si Xiao Wan 232
six bowels 34, 78, 93, 248
six pulses 19
small birth 83
small intestine 52
solid stools 154, 173, 192, 194
somnolence 61, 211
Song Bao Tang 106
Song Zi Dan 94
sore throat 67, 69
spinning head 166
spirit clouding 166
spleen 4-6, 8, 9, 12-15, 28, 29, 34, 38-41, 43, 51, 52, 54-57, 62, 63, 64-67, 69-71, 73, 79, 129, 141, 160, 166, 171, 174, 182, 183, 184, 186, 192, 198, 199, 203, 210-213, 217, 218, 219, 221, 226, 227, 229-231, 233, 234, 248, 252, 255
steaming bone 235, 236, 246
stomach 4-6, 10, 11, 27, 33, 41, 62, 69-71, 73, 78, 88, 113, 123, 124, 128, 136, 137, 141, 142, 152, 153, 158, 166, 182, 184, 188, 190, 192, 202, 203, 208, 209, 213, 215, 218, 219, 221, 229-231, 233, 237, 240, 244, 246, 248, 256
stomach venter 237
strangury 208
sweating 78, 79, 142, 145, 165, 168-171, 173-176, 179, 187, 188, 192, 194, 196-204, 222, 224, 226, 240
swelling & edema in pregnancy 63
swelling and edema of the four limbs 129
swelling of the breasts with red nodules 248
swollen limbs 129

T

tai bing 63
tai dong bu an 66
tai lou 75
tai yang pattern 190
tai yin condition 192
taxation 141, 171, 174, 192, 198, 213, 219, 221, 233, 236, 237, 240, 241
tetany 142, 195, 197
The Treatise on Miscellaneous Conditions 201
thief sweating 201, 202
thirst 10, 24, 25, 61, 78, 79, 86, 122, 162, 170, 171, 179, 192, 194, 196, 200, 203, 204, 214, 222, 223, 250
ti tuo 162
tian gui 38, 55
tiao chan 148
Tiao Gan Tang 44
tiao jing 31, 227
Tiao Jing San 227
Tong Gan Sheng Ru Tang 136
Tong Ru Dan 135
tongue sores 86
toxic swelling 165
transformation of milk 136
transverse delivery 150
transverse presentation 94
treatment methods for the newly birthed 157
trembling 122
triple burner 10, 52
true fire 8, 87, 89
true water 8, 43
two fires 39, 87

U

upper burner 99, 100
urinary bladder 7, 10, 128, 207
urination 10, 11, 162, 165, 201, 203, 208, 209, 229
urination not free 201
uterus 3, 23, 28, 77, 78, 85, 87, 90, 93, 106, 111, 127, 128, 131, 133, 156, 157, 227, 241
uterus-fetus 3

V

vacuity desertion 131, 170, 200
vacuity taxation 240
vagina 10, 53, 132, 245
vaginal discharge disease 4, 9
vanquished form 175
vexation 78, 86, 105, 107, 144, 148, 165, 203, 222, 234
viscera and bowels 26, 64, 113, 219, 221
vomiting 24, 25, 45, 46, 61, 62, 69, 116, 123, 124, 152, 220, 221, 222, 248
vomiting of blood 45, 46, 116

W

wai gan 36
Wan Bao Yin 127
Wan Dai Tang 5
wan gu bu hua 213
Wang Bing 145
wang jian 179
Wang Tai-pu 145
water and grain dysentery 213
water diarrhea 212
water passageway 131
water swelling 64, 130, 218, 226, 227, 255
watery discharge prior to menstruation 51
wei han fu teng xiao chan 88
wei niao 204
wei wan 237
Wen Jing She Xue Tang 34
Wen Qi Hua Shi Tang 47
Wen Wei Ding Xiang San 221
Wen Wei Zhi Ou Tang 124
Wen Zhong Tang 220
wheezing 120
white vaginal discharge 4, 5, 11
widows 4, 21
wind cold 40, 41, 223-225, 237, 241
wound umbilical cord delivery 150, 151
wrenching 3, 21, 26, 27, 73, 74, 85
Wu Ling San 165, 203
Wu Pi San 218, 227
wu po niao bao 207

X

Xi Fen An Tai Tang 79
xia tai 152
xian tian 66, 89
xian tian kidneys 66
xian tian zhi zhen huo 89
xian tian zhi zhen qi 89
xiang huo 80
Xiang Lian Wan 216
xiang sheng 10, 39, 185
xiao chan 83, 85, 86, 88, 90
xiao fu tong 239
Xiao Kuai Tang 166
Xiao Xu Ming Tang 161
Xiao Yao San 7, 37
xie 51, 69, 71, 80, 162, 201, 210, 212-214, 241, 243
xie tong 243
xin chan zhi fa 157
xin tong 237
xing fang xiao chan 83
xing jing hou shao fu teng tong 43
xu lao 240
Xuan Yu Tong Jing Tang 42
xue beng 17, 19, 21, 22, 24, 26, 28, 38, 52, 86, 125, 126, 174, 177, 181
xue beng hun an 17, 19
xue hai da re xue beng 28
xue shi 47, 85
xue xu nan chan 93

Y

yang ming 136, 187, 192, 248
yang ming condition 192
Yang Rong Sheng Hua Tang 232
Yang Rong Zhuang Shen Tang 241
Yang Xin Tang 234
Yang Zheng Tong You Tang 193
yao tong 241
Yellow Emperor 145
yellow facial complexion 26, 49
yellow vaginal discharge 8, 9
Yi Huang Tang 9
Yi Jing 12, 56
Yi Jing Tang 56
Yi Mu Wan 152, 164, 169

Yi Qi Yang Rong Tang 248
Yin Jing Zhi Xue Tang 23
Yin Qi Gui Xue Tang 91
yin tong 244
ying 4, 85, 142, 159, 175, 194, 199, 215, 245
ying and *wei* 159, 199
yu jie xue beng 24
yuan 8, 12, 21, 29, 33, 35, 41, 69, 70, 73, 121, 137, 141, 142, 144, 148, 166, 169, 181, 187, 189, 194, 197, 212, 230, 233, 234, 238, 253
Yuan Tu Gu Tai Tang 70

Z

za zheng 201, 210
Za Zheng Lun 201
(Zhang) Zhong-jing 133, 190
zheng chan 105, 109, 111, 112, 114, 147
zheng chan bai xue gong xin yun kuang 112
zheng chan bao yi bu xia 105
zheng chan chang xia 114
zheng chan qi xu xue yun 109
zheng chan xue yun bu yu 111
zheng chong 233
Zhi Han San 202
zhi xue 17, 22, 23, 25, 26, 76
zhi xue medicinals 76
Zhi Zi Chi Tang 161
Zhu Qi Bu Lou Tang 76
Zhu Xian Dan 37
Zhu Yu Zhi Xue Tang 26
Zhu Zhen-heng 141
Zhuan Qi Tang 130
Zhuan Tian Tang 98
zi gong 28, 156
zi kuang 78
Zi Rong Huo Luo Tang 196
Zi Rong Yang Qi Fu Zheng Tang 188
Zi Rong Yi Qi Fu Shen Tang 172, 181, 182
zi si chan men nan chan 101
zi si fu zhong nan chan 102

OTHER BOOKS ON CHINESE MEDICINE AVAILABLE FROM BLUE POPPY PRESS

1775 Linden Ave
Boulder, CO 80304
For ordering 1-800-487-9296
PH. 303\442-0796 FAX 303\447-0740

PMS: Its Cause, Diagnosis & Treatment According to Traditional Chinese Medicine by Bob Flaws ISBN 0-936185-22-8 $14.95

SOMETHING OLD, SOMETHING NEW; Essays on the TCM Description of Western Herbs, Pharmaceuticals, Vitamins & Minerals by Bob Flaws ISBN 0-936185-21-X $19.95

SCATOLOGY & THE GATE OF LIFE: The Role of the Large Intestine in Immunity, An Integrated Chinese-Western Approach by Bob Flaws ISBN 0-936185-20-1 $12.95

SECOND SPRING: A Guide To Healthy Menopause Through Traditional Chinese Medicine by Honora Lee Wolfe ISBN 0-936185-18-X $14.95

MIGRAINES & TRADITIONAL CHINESE MEDICINE: A Layperson's Guide by Bob Flaws ISBN 0-936185-15-5 $11.95

STICKING TO THE POINT: A Rational Methodology for the Step by Step Formulation & Administration of an Acupuncture Treatment by Bob Flaws ISBN 0-936185-17-1 $14.95

ENDOMETRIOSIS, INFERTILITY AND TRADITIONAL CHINESE MEDICINE: A Laywoman's Guide by Bob Flaws ISBN 0-936185-14-7 $9.95

CLASSICAL MOXIBUSTION SKILLS IN CONTEMPORARY CLINICAL PRACTICE by Sung Baek ISBN 0-936185-16-3 $10.95

THE BREAST CONNECTION: A Laywoman's Guide to the Treatment of Breast Disease by Chinese Medicine by Honora Lee Wolfe ISBN 0-936185-13-9 $8.95

NINE OUNCES: A Nine Part Program For The Prevention of AIDS in HIV Positive Persons by Bob Flaws ISBN 0-936185-12-0 $9.95

THE TREATMENT OF CANCER BY INTEGRATED CHINESE-WESTERN MEDICINE by Zhang Dai-zhao, trans. by Zhang Ting-liang & Bob Flaws, ISBN 0-936185-11-2 $16.95

BLUE POPPY ESSAYS: 1988 Translations and Ruminations on Chinese Medicine by Flaws, Chace et al, ISBN 0-936185-10-4 $18.95

A HANDBOOK OF TRADITIONAL CHINESE DERMATOLOGY by Liang Jian-hui, trans. by Zhang Ting-liang & Bob Flaws, ISBN 0-936185-07-4 $14.95

SECRET SHAOLIN FORMULAE FOR THE TREATMENT OF EXTERNAL INJURY by Patriarch De Chan, trans. by Zhang Ting-liang & Bob Flaws, ISBN 0-936185-08-2 $13.95

A HANDBOOK OF TRADITIONAL CHINESE GYNECOLOGY by Zhejiang College of TCM, trans. by Zhang Ting-liang, ISBN 0-936185-06-6 (2nd edit.) $21.95

FREE & EASY: Traditional Chinese Gynecology for American Women 2nd Edition, by Bob Flaws, ISBN 0-936185-05-8 $15.95

PRINCE WEN HUI'S COOK: Chinese Dietary Therapy by Bob Flaws & Honora Lee Wolfe, ISBN 0-912111-05-4, $12.95 (Published by Paradigm Press, Brookline, MA)

TURTLE TAIL & OTHER TENDER MERCIES: Traditional Chinese Pediatrics by Bob Flaws ISBN 0-936185-00-7 $14.95

THE DAO OF INCREASING LONGEVITY AND CONSERVING ONE'S LIFE by Anna Lin & Bob Flaws, ISBN 0-936185-24-4 $16.95

FIRE IN THE VALLEY: The TCM Diagnosis and Treatment of Vaginal Diseases by Bob Flaws ISBN 0-936185-25-2 $16.95

HIGHLIGHTS OF ANCIENT ACUPUNCTURE PRESCRIPTIONS trans. by Honora Lee Wolfe & Rose Crescenz ISBN 0-936185-23-6 $14.95

ARISAL OF THE CLEAR: A Simple Guide to Healthy Eating According to Traditional Chinese Medicine by Bob Flaws, ISBN #-936185-27-9 $8.95

CERVICAL DYSPLASIA & PROSTATE CANCER: HPV, A HIDDEN LINK? by Bob Flaws, ISBN 0-936185-19-8 $23.95

PEDIATRIC BRONCHITIS: ITS CAUSE, DIAGNOSIS & TREATMENT ACCORDING TO TRADITIONAL CHINESE MEDICINE trans. by Gao Yu-li and Bob Flaws, ISBN 0-936185-26-0 $15.95

AIDS & ITS TREATMENT ACCORDING TO TRADITIONAL CHINESE MEDICINE by Huang Bing-shan, trans. by Fu-Di & Bob Flaws, ISBN 0-936185-28-7 $24.95

ACUTE ABDOMINAL SYNDROMES: Their Diagnosis & Treatment by Combined Chinese-Western Medicine by Alon Marcus DOM, ISBN 0-936185-31-7 $16.95

BEFORE COMPLETION: Essays on the Practice of TCM by Bob Flaws, ISBN 0-936185-32-5

MY SISTER, THE MOON: The Diagnosis & Treatment of Menstrual Diseases by Traditional Chinese Medicine by Bob Flaws, ISBN 0-936185-34-1, $24.95

FU QING-ZHU'S GYNECOLOGY trans. by Yang Shou-zhong and Liu Da-wei, ISBN 0-936185-35-X, $21.95

FLESHING OUT THE BONES: The Importance of Case Histories in Chinese Medicine trans. by Charles Chace. ISBN 0-936185-30-9, $18.95